The
Healthcare
Leader's
GUIDE
to
Actions,
Awareness,
and Perception

The
Healthcare
Leader's
GUIDE
to
Actions,
Awareness,
and Perception

THIRD EDITION

Carson F. Dye and Brett D. Lee

ACHE Management Series

Your board, staff, or clients may also benefit from this book's insight. For more information on quantity discounts, contact the Health Administration Press Marketing Manager at (312) 424-9450.

This publication is intended to provide accurate and authoritative information in regard to the subject matter covered. It is sold, or otherwise provided, with the understanding that the publisher is not engaged in rendering professional services. If professional advice or other expert assistance is required, the services of a competent professional should be sought.

The statements and opinions contained in this book are strictly those of the authors and do not represent the official positions of the American College of Healthcare Executives or the Foundation of the American College of Healthcare Executives.

20   5   4   3   2

Library of Congress Cataloging-in-Publication Data
Names: Dye, Carson F., author. | Lee, Brett D., author.
Title: The healthcare leader's guide to actions, awareness, and perception / Carson F. Dye and Brett D. Lee.
Other titles: Executive excellence (Health Administration Press)
Description: Third edition. | Chicago, Illinois : Health Administration Press, 2016. | Revision of: Executive excellence / Carson F. Dye. 2nd ed. c2000. | Includes index.
Identifiers: LCCN 2015038823| ISBN 9781567937657 (print : alk. paper) | ISBN 9781567937664 (epub) | ISBN 9781567937671 (mobi) | ISBN 9781567937862 (vbk) | ISBN 9781567937879 (xml) | ISBN 9781567937886 (ebook)
Subjects: LCSH: Health services administrators—Conduct of life. | Business etiquette.
Classification: LCC RA971 .D94 2016 | DDC 362.1068/4—dc23 LC record available at http://lccn.loc.gov/2015038823

The paper used in this publication meets the minimum requirements of American National Standard for Information Sciences—Permanence of Paper for Printed Library Materials, ANSI Z39.48-1984. ∞ ™

Acquisitions editor: Janet Davis; Project manager: Michael Noren; Cover designer: Brad Norr; Layout: PerfecType

Found an error or a typo? We want to know! Please e-mail it to hapbooks@ache.org, and put "Book Error" in the subject line.

For photocopying and copyright information, please contact Copyright Clearance Center at www.copyright.com or at (978) 750-8400.

Health Administration Press
A division of the Foundation of the American
    College of Healthcare Executives
300 S. Riverside Plaza, Suite 1900
Chicago, IL 60606-6698
(312) 424-2800

In memory of two wonderful leaders who have gone forward to a higher road:

Edward J. Arlinghaus, PhD, Xavier University health services administration program chair from 1966 to 1992, whose "Arlinghaus-O-Grams" inspired my first *Protocols* book in 1993;

and

Kenneth H. Cohn, MD, author, teacher, learner, surgeon, friend, and valued colleague, whose spirit represented the pinnacles of how to conduct oneself and inspire others to be more gracious and respectful.

C.F.D.

I would like to dedicate this book to my wife, Mindy, and son, Preston, for being the steady foundation in my life, the source of inspiration, and the reason for more smiles than I can count.

B.D.L.

Contents

Part III   Serving Inside the Organization

Part IV   Capstone

Foreword

ASK YOURSELF THIS: How often do you think about your professional image, and do you purposefully manage it as one of your most valuable assets?

Image, reputation, and personal brand can make or break a career in healthcare, yet these elements continue to be overlooked or poorly understood by so many otherwise qualified leaders. In *The Healthcare Leader's Guide to Actions, Awareness, and Perception*, Carson Dye and Brett Lee provide valuable insights into these key aspects of leadership and provide practical advice for enhancing self-awareness and avoiding costly career missteps.

Carson is one of the top executive recruiters and leadership gurus in the United States. He has an uncanny knack—a laserlike insight, a deep intuitive sense—for what makes some leaders succeed and others fail, and it's this highly refined understanding that makes his books so uniquely compelling and valuable. This book isn't like all the other leadership titles lining the shelves of your favorite bookstore; frankly, it's in a class all its own.

For this third edition of the book, Carson has taken on Brett Lee as a coauthor, in part to lend a more youthful perspective to the topic. Note, however, that Brett's youth should not be mistaken for inexperience: Brett has accomplished much in his 15 years in healthcare, having won an impressive array of awards and honors and having already served in executive roles at some of the nation's largest pediatric hospitals.

Over the course of my own career, Carson has been a trusted friend and colleague. He's the best career coach I know. Many times I have said to him after a conversation or after reading a book he just gave me, "I wish I had known that at the beginning of my career." Well, I'm feeling that same way once again: *The Healthcare Leader's Guide to Actions, Awareness, and Perception* is a book I wish I had read when I was younger, because it would have saved me from a number of blunders in my quest to refine my executive presence.

Perhaps like you, I didn't have the benefit of a mentor or a wise sage early in my career. I was never taught the importance of self-awareness and perception. If I had known back then what I know now after reading Carson and Brett's book, my road to the executive suite would have been much smoother. Sadly, I've seen many promising careers derailed—some temporarily and others permanently—by missteps that could have been avoided with this book's teachings.

Carson and Brett have a writing style that is straightforward, clear, and concise. There's no fluff; everything is relevant and immensely practical. Healthcare leaders at every career stage— seasoned executives, people just starting in administrative roles, and everyone in between—will be well served by the protocols contained in this book.

We all have that special bookshelf in our office where we keep our most valued books. You know the ones—the books we've read over and over, the ones filled with highlights, notes, and dog-eared pages. *The Healthcare Leader's Guide to Actions, Awareness, and Perception* definitely deserves a place at the head of that row.

John Byrnes, MD
President and CEO
Byrnes Group LLC
Grand Rapids, Michigan

Preface

THIS BOOK MAY literally save your career. That surely is a dramatic statement—perhaps arrogant, perhaps overstated, perhaps over the top. Yet we strongly believe that the insights contained herein will heighten self-awareness for some readers to the point that they change problematic behavior before a career-ending event.

The lesson of the book is simple: As a leader, you have a responsibility to be aware of how you are perceived and to act appropriately. Appropriate action applies to behavior, conduct, courtesy, ethics, professional demeanor, dress, and respect. Some of the guidelines presented in this book could fall under the realm of emotional intelligence. However, this book's protocols extend beyond emotional intelligence and cover many aspects of leadership that can make or break a career.

In brief, this book is based on the following precepts:

- As a leader, you are highly visible, and others constantly watch you—often very closely. The ways others perceive you will have a significant impact on your success or failure. The saying that "perception can be more important than reality" is operative in a very real way.
- Organizations, and society in general, have many unwritten rules and expectations for leaders, and they are different from and often more rigorous than the rules and expectations for the rank and file.

- Once leaders become more advanced in their careers and move higher up in their organizations, they are likely to be evaluated primarily on organizational measures of success (e.g., quality or financial results, physician satisfaction, patient experience, employee engagement). In contrast, leaders early in their careers are likely to receive direct feedback about their behaviors and the perceptions of others, often in the form of mentoring. As leaders become more mature in their positions, they receive less feedback. As this trend continues, experienced leaders can easily lose touch with the ways that unwritten rules and expectations affect them. Furthermore, feedback of a personal nature can often be most distressful to senior leaders. Uncomfortable confrontations and awkward discussions can sometimes bring to mind the Hans Christian Andersen fable of the emperor with no clothes.

- A leader's key competencies can be grouped into five categories: (1) leadership competencies, such as well-cultivated self-awareness, compelling vision, masterful execution, and a real way with people (Dye and Garman 2015); (2) technical attributes and specialized knowledge related to specific positions (e.g., accounting principles for chief financial officers, care management for nursing leaders, labor and employment laws for human resources leaders); (3) administrative abilities, such as organizational skill, time management, meeting management, and prioritization; (4) human resources matters, often related to employee interactions and conflict resolution; and (5) appropriateness of behavior, anchored by self-awareness, ethics, and understanding of proper conduct. This book focuses on the fifth category.

The field of executive coaching is growing rapidly, and we believe that much of its growth is correlated with a heightened awareness of the need for guidance and feedback at every level of leadership. The lessons in this book are appropriate for all leaders, whether they are in the early, middle, or late stages of their careers:

- *Early-career leaders.* Academic leaders from a number of health administration graduate programs have asked for resources to guide students going into fellowships or full-time jobs and to help students better understand the nature of the working world. People who are new to executive meeting rooms and boardrooms often lack a firm understanding of how they are perceived, and young leaders often allow an early taste of authority to create stumbling blocks. This book can help leaders avoid those early-career missteps.

- *Midcareer leaders.* Much academic literature about managerial derailment speaks to the problems encountered by leaders who spend 15 to 20 years growing and advancing in their careers, only to develop problems and ultimately derail. This book aims to reinforce self-awareness and help leaders keep their careers on track.

- *Late-career leaders.* Many seasoned leaders fail to receive sufficient feedback and constructive criticism, and some allow the trappings of power and status to cloud their judgment. This book can guide them as they develop ongoing feedback mechanisms to let them know how they are truly perceived.

The first edition of this book was published by Health Administration Press in 1993 and carried the title *Protocols for Health Care Executive Behavior: A Factor for Success.* Over the more than 20 years of the book's history, many readers have commented on the book's usefulness, its application, and the unique but common-sense nature of its message. This third edition, with the title revised to *The Healthcare Leader's Guide to Actions, Awareness, and Perception,* may capture that message best of all, thanks in part to a new coauthor who represents the next generation of leaders.

Please read the book with an open mind and a willingness to step up your self-awareness. It may save your career.

Carson F. Dye
Brett D. Lee

REFERENCE

Dye, C. F., and A. N. Garman. 2015. *Exceptional Leadership: 16 Critical Competencies for Healthcare Executives*, 2nd ed. Chicago: Health Administration Press.

Acknowledgments

THIS THIRD EDITION represents my tenth book, all with Health Administration Press, and I begin my acknowledgments with them—the publisher, the partner, the organization that provides us with such great learning material in our field. The entire staff at HAP is exemplary and exceptional. Special thanks to Janet Davis, who is positively inspiring and always pushing us to "build a better mousetrap." I had other books I wanted to write, but Janet was persuasive in telling me of the demand for a fresher version of this one. I am also very appreciative of our editor, Michael Noren, who put the final spit and polish on the book. Michael reminds me of another Michael in Chicago, and I think this one (Mr. Noren) has similarities of skill level to the basketball Michael. He certainly made this manuscript richer and more meaningful. I have said it before and will repeat it again: Health Administration Press continues to provide outstanding tools for those of us in the healthcare field.

The first two editions of this book were solo works. Staring at the possibility of a third edition made me think that a partner would be in order. Aware that many healthcare leaders are from a generation different from my own, I looked for someone who was more representative of the great up-and-coming leadership ranks in our field—and there appeared Brett Lee. Frankly, I did not know that he had been one of *Modern Healthcare* magazine's 2013 "Up and Comers" when Janet Davis suggested that the two of us talk. It did not take long for me to realize that he had a hunger for leadership growth and that he shared my beliefs about the little things that can make or break our careers as leaders. He has brought fresh ideas to the book and ensured that we have some viewpoints that are not from the gray-haired crowd. Brett brought new life to the original material and has been a great partner in this endeavor.

Many of our chapters have guest commentaries, in which the book's essential themes are approached by respected colleagues with diverse points of view. I thank and acknowledge all the individuals who took the time to review our material, draft commentaries, and share them with us:

Jeremy C. Adams
Timothy P. Adams
Kelvin A. Baggett
Kenneth H. Cohn
J. Eric Evans
Gerry Ibay
John "Jack" R. Janoso, Jr.
Scott A. Malaney
Bill McLean
J. Mark McLoone
Britt T. Reynolds
Michelle Taylor Smith
Joe Thomason

Over the past 22 years, my consulting and leadership-search work has brought me into contact with hundreds of wonderful healthcare leaders. I am indebted to all of them for their stories, contributions, and experiences. The depth of knowledge that has been given to me is vast, and it has shaped many of the ideas and precepts in this book. Some special leaders stand out in the crowd and have served as role models for my thinking and leadership reflections. I include in that list Scott Malaney, Chip Hubbs, Dr. Frank Byrne, Dr. John Byrnes, Dr. Lee Hammerling, Dr. Mark

Laney, Dr. Scott Ransom, Dr. Kathleen Forbes, Dr. Greg Taylor, the late Dr. Ken Cohn, Tom Beeman, Michael Covert, Kyle Campbell, David Rubenstein, Cynthia Moore-Hardy, Randy Oostra, and Randy Schimmoeller.

I close with my family. I have been truly blessed by them, and I count them as very special influencers. I am very lucky to have them.

C.F.D.

I would like to thank Carson Dye for inviting me to help reintroduce his thoughts to a new generation of healthcare leaders. It has been a great deal of fun working with you!

Special thanks to Janet Davis, Health Administration Press, and the American College of Healthcare Executives for your support.

B.D.L.

Introduction

*Bosses—especially senior ones—overestimate the significance
of their routine decision making and underestimate
the impact of their personal behavior.*

—Walter F. Ulmer, Jr.

WHAT IS IMPLIED by the phrase *leadership success*? How is such
success measured or determined? What contributes to the success
of senior managers and executives who are recognized as being at
the top of their field?

Generally, successful leaders in healthcare are those people
deemed to be personally responsible for successful organizations—
those organizations that have strong financial bottom lines, excellent reputations within their communities, high-quality and loyal
medical staffs, and substantial market share. Are the executives
really personally responsible for these organizational hallmarks? In
many cases, they are.

THE SENSE OF THE APPROPRIATE

Successful leaders have numerous skills and attributes that contribute to their success. This book will address in detail one of the

most important—the "sense of the appropriate." Skilled executives and senior managers understand the importance of appropriate personal behavior and relationships and are aware of the negative effect that offensive, peculiar, or eccentric behavior can have upon achievements. They practice "executive etiquette." They know the principles of courtesy, their personal standards are proper, and their ethics are beyond reproach. Most successful leaders are conscious of their own personality and behavior quirks, and they work hard at preventing them from undermining the sense of the appropriate.

Of course, some executives may exhibit annoying or offensive habits and behavior and still achieve success, as measured by traditional organizational gauges. However, such executives are in the minority; it is rare to find successful executives who are not accomplished at understanding their own behavior and controlling it in a socially (and institutionally) acceptable fashion.

Unfortunately, no established codes of conduct govern all the various behavioral expectations in business, and no set of rules or standards can cover every possible situation leaders encounter. However, our society does have certain principles that determine socially acceptable behavior. Some of these principles are very clear, but others are not. Senior managers and executives should be aware of these societal principles and the need to follow them.

This book does not purport to set forth appropriate behavior protocols for every situation that senior managers will confront. The reader will always have to exercise judgment and keep a sense of perspective when confronted with issues in the workplace. Still, we hope the discussions in this book will serve as a kind of "mirror" to help readers reflect upon and gain a better understanding of their behavior. The book is an appeal to all healthcare leaders to realize that a sense of the appropriate is an extremely important element of successful management and leadership.

Readers will undoubtedly say, "This is merely good common sense." Some will think, "I already know this—why am I reading this?" Some seasoned executives may remain aloof from and untouched by the book's messages. Others may believe the messages are too conceptual and philosophical to be practical. However, a large number of executives have read the manuscript and reinforced the concepts behind it. They have shared many "war stories," some of which are used as examples in the book. The fact is that a number of healthcare executives have had less-than-successful tenures within their organizations because they had a poor understanding of the need for appropriate behavior or were unwilling to change their behavior. Some have lost their jobs for these reasons.

Within the healthcare world, the word *protocol* has a rich and deep meaning. It typically refers to the commonly accepted way of doing things to and for patients. The protocol is the right way—the way most professionals do things. Many medical protocols are not written in any codified manner but rather passed on from one generation of physicians to another, often during medical rounds. Our hope is that this book can serve as an administrative grand rounds to help the reader comprehend the significance of behavioral issues. The intent is to help the reader develop a sense of the appropriate.

Executive search consultants can relate countless stories of senior-level candidates who are technically proficient and have great careers but find their progress interrupted because of seemingly minor incidents or slight personal idiosyncrasies. The following are just a few examples of how managers and executives can lose their effectiveness or, worse yet, their positions because of inappropriate behavior:

- The director of one of the leading graduate programs in health administration received a phone call one Monday morning from a star alumnus who had graduated three years earlier. In those days (the early 1970s), an MHA graduate typically entered a healthcare organization as an assistant administrator and could expect a relatively rapid move up the hospital corporate ladder.

This former student was on the fast track as an assistant administrator at his first hospital and was about to be promoted to the number-two position under the top administrator. That Monday morning, however, he was asked by his chief executive officer to find a new job. Apparently, the former student had attended a party on Saturday night at the home of the president of the medical staff, had a few too many drinks, and told offensive jokes while wrapping his arm around the shoulders of the medical staff president's wife. The formerly up-and-coming young executive was told by the CEO that his behavior had greatly embarrassed the medical staff president and that several other physicians had expressed disapproval. Thus, the CEO continued, the young man's credibility had been damaged and it was unlikely that he could be successful at the institution. He was given six months to find another job.

After the graduate program director hung up the phone, he reflected on the performance and behavior of this alumnus while he was in school. The program chair recalled occasions in which the rest of the graduate class talked of this student's "weekend drunks" and tendency to "party." The warning signs of future problems were apparent even then. Although this young man was an excellent student and had good interpersonal skills on a day-to-day basis, his one vice cost him greatly. The chair of the graduate program wishes to this day that he had heeded the warning signs and intervened while this individual was still in school. Perhaps this humiliating and damaging experience could have been avoided.

- An unmarried CEO had all of the managerial tickets and was running his organization quite successfully. After a few years, he began dating the ex-wife of a former hospital board member. Although the two were open about their relationship, the ex-husband became incensed and led a movement to replace the CEO. The ensuing struggle split the board of directors and the medical staff, and it harmed the hospital for a number of years. The CEO eventually left the organization because of the controversy.

- A vice president of professional services was twice passed over for promotion to a chief operating officer (COO) position. The reason was simple: Several members of the medical staff had petitioned the CEO, each time indicating that they felt that the vice president's past personal relationships with several of the nurse managers would harm his effectiveness. Although the medical staff were comfortable with him in the professional services role, they did not want to see him move higher into the COO position.

Readers should keep an open mind as they move through this book. They should not be too quick to say, "That's not me." Rather, they should use the book for motivation as they strive to uncover character flaws and idiosyncrasies that might undermine their effectiveness and professional success. Without constant vigilance and self-awareness, one can all too easily forget the sense of the appropriate. The descriptions of problem behavior found in this book can fit many of us, at one time or another.

HOW THIS BOOK IS STRUCTURED

The book is divided into three parts. Part I, "Managing Yourself—Self-Discipline," introduces the concept of protocols. We aim to provide a model for executive success that centers on the concept of appropriate leadership behavior. The underlying principle suggests that character and values drive behavior and thus can be the underlying foundations for the practice of appropriate behavior. Chapters 1 through 5 focus on specific areas of individual behavior.

Part II, "Serving Others," sets forth a number of principles about how leaders should interact with others. Implicit throughout is the belief that a new form of leadership, that of "servant leadership," can become a strong pathway to personal success. Chapters 6 through 12 provide specific guides in critical areas of focus.

Part III, "Serving Inside the Organization," examines the various ways leadership behavior can be important within the context of the larger organization. Of particular importance are the chapters that address protocols relating to cultural diversity and men and women in the workplace. Chapters 13 through 16 offer specific insight on appropriate leadership behavior in these areas.

Finally, Chapter 17 serves as a capstone to focus in on two critical issues that surround this entire book—self-awareness and derailment.

This book cannot possibly cover every situation that healthcare leaders are likely to encounter. However, the examples provided should help acquaint readers with the basic principles of appropriate executive behavior and how they apply in actual practice.

A WORD ABOUT THE TITLE

Earlier we spoke of the word *protocol*. The title of the first edition of this book, published in 1993, was *Protocols for Health Care Executive Behavior: A Factor for Success*. The original conceptual model suggested that there were four factors that contributed to the success of executives, and the factors were presented in a formula:

Executive Success =
Effective Technical Skills and Knowledge
× Administrative Skills and Knowledge
× Human Resources Skills and Knowledge
× Appropriate Executive Behavior ("Protocols")

The text stated: "Note that the formula is a multiplicative function with four factors; a zero in any of the factors results in a zero product—zero executive success. . . . The lack of or weakness in any one of these four factors will minimize executive success, whereas strength in these areas will enhance success." The second edition, published in 2000 and titled *Executive Excellence: Protocols for Healthcare Leaders*, continued this theme.

At the time of the first two editions, very few books focused on the *personal* aspects of leadership. Instead, most leadership books presented topics pertaining to team building, developing vision and strategy, and organizational management. They were *organizational* in nature. The *Protocols* books sold well over the years and gained a following. It is certainly hoped that many careers were helped along the way.

The title of this third edition, *The Healthcare Leader's Guide to Actions, Awareness, and Perception*, represents an intensified look at certain aspects and a more modern focus in some respects, but the idea and early concept of protocols remain.

PART I

Managing Yourself—Self-Discipline

CHAPTER 1

Perception Versus Reality

*It is very difficult to manage your way out of a situation that
your behavior has gotten you into.*

—Stephen Covey

Guide to Reader

This chapter forms a critical foundation for the leadership
precepts in this book. It centers on the principle that
leaders must be aware of how they are perceived *and* be
willing to change behavior if a need to do so is indicated.
Rooted in self-awareness, the ability to understand how you
are perceived forms the underpinning for all highly effective
leadership. Essentially, the message of this chapter—and
this book—is that perception is more important than reality
and one of the principal jobs of leaders is to discern how
they are perceived.

Actions Louder Than Words

The CEO of a large academic medical center took great pride in being a visible leader within his organization and in personally championing key strategic initiatives with the frontline staff. The latest endeavor that he and his executive team were looking to achieve was a reduction of nosocomial infections by 50 percent in 12 months, with an ultimate goal of eliminating all preventable hospital-acquired infections within three years. The chairman of the board of trustees led a hospital-wide kickoff for the initiative with a great deal of fanfare, and the laudable goal was touted in a series of town hall meetings hosted by the CEO. An aggressive staff training and internal marketing campaign was developed and initiated. A key component of the implementation involved "patient safety rounds," which were designed to make senior leaders more visible in the organization, to engage frontline staff in a dialogue about the enhanced focus on infection prevention, and to track progress on unit-specific tactics and goals associated with the program. The CEO was particularly excited about this aspect of the initiative, as it centered on his self-perceived strengths of building effective relationships with staff and leveraging those relationships to create enthusiasm toward a strategic goal. He began performing his rounds daily with a great deal of fervor, and he felt he was gaining a great deal of support with the staff while increasing awareness of infection prevention. The CEO thus was surprised when the chief nursing officer requested a private meeting a few weeks later to discuss some complaints she had received about the patient safety rounds. She carefully began the discussion by telling the CEO that, although the staff

(continued)

(continued from previous page)

greatly appreciated his visits and his enthusiasm toward the goal of creating a safer environment for patients, they were concerned that he had been witnessed several times entering and exiting patient rooms without performing proper hand hygiene. Moreover, his habit of shaking the hands or patting the backs of employees to make personal connections while rounding could actually be a detriment to the goals that he was holding them personally accountable to achieve. The feedback provided the CEO with a powerful reminder of the disconnect that existed between his internally held image of his activities and the very different perception he was creating with the frontline staff.

Be mindful: In the case of leaders, our actions form stronger impressions with those whom we lead than our words ever could. And remember the old adage: Perception is often more important than reality.

LEADERSHIP: THE MOST IMPORTANT REALITY WE HAVE IS HOW WE ARE PERCEIVED

In healthcare, leadership is, at its core, a business of building and maintaining positive relationships. And a leader's ability to develop effective relationships with peers, subordinates, and supervisors is greatly influenced by the perceptions people form during inter-actions. Just as a photograph can capture a moment in time and reinforce that moment in our memories, personal interactions with leaders in an organization can shape our perceptions of the leaders' personality, character, and ability to lead. These impressions can be lasting, and they have the potential to either enhance or destroy the careers of technically capable leaders.

Sadly, a gap often exists between how leaders perceive themselves and how they are viewed by those they have been invited to lead, and this gap tends to widen as executives take on more senior roles. Lombardo and Eichinger (2002) found that, when completing self-assessments in 360-degree performance reviews, leaders tended to rate themselves an average of .75 point higher on a five-point scale than their subordinates rated them. Lombardo and Eichinger also found that the most senior executives were increasingly likely to overrate themselves, particularly in the area of

---

Leadership Research and Theory Support

Much of the evidential research on the need for leaders to understand how they are perceived comes from the field of psychology. The term *confirmation bias*, used in psychological literature, describes the tendency for individuals to interpret evidence so that it is in accordance with their own beliefs. Leaders must be aware of this bias. Nickerson's (1998) writing on the topic is complex but worth reviewing.

> Nickerson, R. S. 1998. "Confirmation Bias: A Ubiquitous Phenomenon in Many Guises." *Review of General Psychology* 2 (2): 175–220.

Knight (2011) writes: "Unmanaged perception becomes a truth that was not intended. So, as leaders if you want to communicate successfully, influence, or lead people, you must understand how you are perceived so you can change perception."

> Knight, P. 2011. "Leaders: How Do You Manage Perception?" Blog. Published April 18. http://patriciaknight.wordpress.com/2011/04/18/leaders-how-do-you-manage-perception/.

(continued)

(continued from previous page)

An additional area supported by research is self-awareness. Self-awareness is simply the ability to view oneself introspectively and put that observation to use in improving interpersonal relationships. According to Fletcher and Bailey (2003), increasing self-awareness is thought to enhance performance. Most will agree that an increased level of self-awareness will enhance a leader's ability to understand the perceptions of others.

Fletcher, C., and C. Bailey. 2003. "Assessing Self-Awareness: Some Issues and Methods." *Journal of Managerial Psychology* 18 (5): 395–404.

emotional intelligence. Furthermore, senior executives were found to be less likely to have reliable mechanisms for gaining feedback on their professional performance and potential areas for continued development.

Significant gaps can exist because of the distance, both real and perceived, between executives in an organization and the front-line staff. Despite trends toward a more relaxed work environment and the empowerment of employees, executives remain foreboding figures in the healthcare field. Consequently, executives are not often challenged by their employees and, even worse, are not openly criticized or offered suggestions for personal or professional improvement. Even when outspoken employees do challenge executives, those leaders often will retreat to the privacy and safety of their offices, and the duty of responding will be delegated to lower-ranking executives. In seeking shelter from the realities of the organization, executives can skew their perceptions of the needs and sentiments of employees and develop falsely positive impressions of their own performance as leader.

The distance between executives and employees only widens the perception gap because (1) it creates two differing perceptions of reality and (2) employees misunderstand, and possibly get offended by, executives' lack of insight into issues within the organization. The bottom line in this situation is that people believe what they perceive to be true, even if there may be valid evidence to the contrary (see the note on confirmation bias in this chapter's "Leadership Research and Theory Support" box). An executive may be able to produce objective financial results, but the results may be of little consequence if the executive fails to capture the hearts and minds of those who work for him.

Lack of organizational self-awareness can be significantly detrimental to long-term success. A study that followed a group of executives longitudinally over time to track their career progression found that leaders who rated themselves significantly more favorably than other rater groups did on core leadership competencies also failed to recognize potential career-stalling behaviors. Those leaders were also more likely to be terminated than peers who had a view of their own performance that was more aligned with other rating groups in the 360-degree evaluation (Lombardo and Eichinger 2003). Findings from the study are shown in Exhibit 1.1.

EXHIBIT 1.1: Career Progressions Associated with Self-Rating Scores Significantly More Favorable Than Other Rater Scores

Measure	Terminated	Unchanged	Promoted
Self-rated higher on leadership competencies	30	22	1
Self-rated higher on career-stalling behaviors	10	6	0
Total self-rating more favorable	40	28	1

Source: Reprinted with permission from Lombardo and Eichinger (2003).

What does this mean? Simply put, the responsibility for recognizing and managing perception lies solely on the executive. Consider the following case examples:

- An executive in charge of an organization-wide strategic project spoke frequently with her team in both individual and group settings about her personal commitment to the initiative. When business conditions changed, however, she began to divert attention and budget funding away from the project without explaining the rationale to her team. In the absence of information from their leader, the team came to the conclusion that she was not supporting them adequately, and they worried that their continued participation in the project might derail their own careers in the organization. The project ground to a halt, and trust in the leader was irrevocably lost.

- A hospital CEO was active in a number of local community organizations. He believed that his community service was providing excellent visibility for his organization and that his involvement was fully supported by the board. After his resignation, however, the committee in charge of finding his replacement gave the executive search firm clear instructions that they wanted a CEO who would spend more time in the hospital and less time with the Chamber of Commerce, Rotary Club, and other groups.

- A dynamic new vice president was brought into an organization and quickly began trying to make a name for herself. She made rapid changes in staffing, leadership structure, and service offerings and did so somewhat unilaterally. Although she delivered financial gains for the company as a result of her restructuring, she failed to recognize that the historical organizational culture was one of collaboration and consensus building. Peers were so angered by her lack of communication and her "empire building" that she was eventually forced out of the organization.

- Because of a sustained downward trend in volumes and revenues, a hospital CEO announced in a series of town hall meetings that everyone needed to pitch in and "tighten their belts" and that there would be a salary freeze and a significant reduction in force to rebase expenses going forward. Shortly after the layoffs were completed, the local paper published a story on the sizable bonuses that the hospital executive team had been paid for improving the organization's financial performance. Obviously, the news created a great deal of negative sentiment among the staff.

These case examples are similar because they all revolve around half-truths and perceptions formed in the absence of effective communication on the part of the executives. To avoid situations of this type, leaders must understand the common causes of misperception, work to develop self-awareness, ensure that they have a process to recognize and change poor perceptions in the organization, and establish mechanisms to foster positive ongoing perceptions.

COMMON CAUSES OF POOR LEADERSHIP PERCEPTION

Employees can form misperceptions about their leaders based on a wide variety of factors. However, certain factors have proved to be common triggers and must be actively managed by executives looking to maintain a positive image within the organization. Leaders must be aware that they are always "on stage" and that their actions are being judged at every moment. The list of factors discussed here is far from exhaustive, but it highlights how certain words and symbols associated with positions of authority can easily be misconstrued. Such misunderstandings can call into question the motives and integrity of leaders who are not mindful of crafting their organizational identity.

Executive Compensation

The Great Recession of 2007–2009 brought renewed attention to the issue of executive compensation—a historically touchy subject and something that continues to draw a great deal of ire from frontline employees today. Stories about corporate CEOs taking large executive bonuses while their companies faltered contributed to the "Occupy Wall Street" movement, and revelations that Wal-Mart CEO Michael Duke made more in one hour than the average Wal-Mart employee earned in a year sparked national outrage (Gomstyn 2010). Compensation of healthcare leaders, though not at the level of *Fortune* 500 CEOs, has also been the focus of criticism during healthcare reform debates. Some states have placed caps on income levels for CEOs of not-for-profit providers. In addition, a new Securities and Exchange Commission (2015) rule requires publicly traded hospitals to publish the ratio of their CEOs' total compensation to the median employee compensation—a response to increasing public concern over the gap between CEO pay and employee pay.

Healthcare leaders must be sensitive to the fact that their compensation packages are often much higher than those of frontline staff. And even though a competitive compensation strategy is critical to retaining top-level leadership talent, the methods of determining those compensation levels (market surveys, board-level recommendations) are often poorly understood by the rank and file of the organization. Likewise, much of the work an executive does occurs out of the line of sight of the staff, and staff might not always fully appreciate the strategic decisions executives make to ensure the long-term sustainability of the organization. Leaders must understand this dynamic, be keenly aware not to flaunt the "trappings of success," and remember that they are being scrutinized. Actions as seemingly innocuous as decorating your office lavishly or having a hallway discussion about purchasing a new sports car can serve to create a rift—the best leaders understand this innate tension and actively work to manage it.

Perquisites

Another common source of negative perception involves perquisites, or perks—the tangible representations of the value the company has placed on its leader. Company cars (or car allowances), reserved parking spaces, social club memberships, and posh executive dining areas are among the perks seen in some areas of healthcare. Even the simplest of catered business lunches in the hospital administrative suite cause some eyebrows to rise. Highly visible perks, although desirable and almost expected with senior-level positions in an organization, can host a litany of problems, including the following:

- *Bitterness over imbalance of power.* Leaders need to understand that there are likely employees within the organization who feel they work harder than, are at least as well qualified as, and are equally deserving of success as their executives. The visibility of perks can serve as a discernible trigger to this subset of employees and lead to insubordination and low employee morale.
- *Financial and quality ramifications.* Once a few employees get infected with the wrong perception, that same way of thinking can spread to a larger group of employees quickly and easily. Results of this viral spread may include lower staff productivity, slipping of key quality and operational metrics, and negative long-term effects on the bottom line.

Perks are an important part of a competitive compensation package and are often necessary for the recruitment of talented candidates. However, leaders must recognize and manage the way employees perceive these perks. Leaders should exercise care in taking advantage of perks that might be considered inappropriate given the unique culture of the organization or the specific conditions at the time. For instance, a CEO driving an expensive sports car into a reserved parking space might cause significant strain on staff relations, especially if it occurs during a time when the hospital is struggling financially and focusing on expense and job cutting.

Leadership Visibility

One of the most common criticisms of leaders in healthcare is that they are rarely seen in the operations of the hospital. No matter how often a leader rounds or walks through the facility, some employees still would like to see her more often. Most healthcare organizations operate on a 24-hours-a-day, 7-days-a-week cycle, so even if an executive spends a great deal of time getting to know the staff on the day shift, the night shift might feel alienated. This dynamic only becomes more pronounced as leaders move up in an organization or move to organizations of greater size and scale. The simple truth is that most employees in a healthcare setting are caregivers by nature, and relationships play an important role in their sense of job satisfaction. If employees do not feel they have an effective working relationship with their direct supervisor, and if they do not feel connected to their senior leaders, the likelihood of them seeking employment elsewhere will be significantly higher.

Less-visible executives often develop both real and perceived distances from frontline employees, are perceived as aloof or uncaring, and have a weak grasp of the day-to-day issues in the organization. Regardless of competing priorities, it is imperative that leaders at all levels carve out specific time on a regular basis to spend in the operations; to speak with staff about the direction of the organization, key goals, and metrics the staff can influence; and to actively seek feedback about how leaders can help staff perform their jobs more effectively. Senior executives should round not only during the day shift but also periodically during evenings and weekends (ideally these responsibilities can be distributed to each executive team member on a rotating basis). Other methods to enhance leadership visibility may include regular town hall meetings and informal breakfast sessions with employees celebrating their anniversary months with the organization.

EFFECTIVELY MANAGING NEGATIVE PERCEPTIONS

To effectively manage perception, executives must develop an understanding of leadership that includes a grasp of how their behavior influences the environment around them. Through daily contact with supervisors, peers, and subordinates, a personal leadership profile is constructed one interaction at a time. Effective leadership requires a high level of self-awareness that enhances knowledge of personal strengths and weaknesses. It also requires the adoption of a process for effectively responding to and turning around negative perceptions that may have developed. The protocol displayed in Exhibit 1.2 and described in the sections that follow provides an effective framework:

EXHIBIT 1.2: Protocol for Managing Perception

Because implication does not equal inference, executives must ensure that everyone receives the intended messages and meanings by

1. recognizing the perception,
2. discovering the genesis of the perception,
3. actively changing or correcting the perception, and
4. reinforcing and maintaining the appropriate perception.

Recognize the Perception

Pretending that a misunderstanding is not happening will not make it go away. You should acknowledge it without personalizing it and develop an action plan to remedy it.

Discover the Genesis of the Perception

Find out through research or by asking people directly how the issue began. Do not veil your efforts or pit one employee against another. You should not seek to justify your viewpoint or recruit others to your perspective; doing so may only serve to multiply the wrong impression.

Actively Change or Correct the Perception

The only way to address an issue is to face it, so talk to the people involved and offer an explanation or apology if needed. Change behaviors that were the root of the issue and make sure you inform others of your efforts to change. Such matters are best handled personally, as delegating apologies tends to lessen the impact. Also, e-mail is rarely the best method for this type of communication. Your personal effort in correcting the matter is the quickest way to convince people that you care.

Reinforce and Maintain the Good Perception

Keep the people who work with you and for you informed and invested in the truth; doing so will make misunderstandings less pervasive. Remember the common causes of poor leadership perception, and actively manage frequently misinterpreted words and symbols.

The framework in Exhibit 1.2 may seem intuitive. However, putting these concepts into practice may prove more difficult than anticipated due to the time, energy, and humility involved in reversing negative perceptions. Changing an existing perception does not happen overnight, as that perception has often been based on multiple instances of observed behavior on the part of the executive. The perception is likely to endure until the staff sees the executive demonstrating new behavior in a repeated fashion over an extended period of time.

Unfortunately, many executives do not practice any type of protocol when managing employee perception. Amazingly, some simply seem to be unaware. These executives do not follow up on issues that have surfaced from frontline staff because, in the executives' minds, accountability to subordinate employees decreases as their accountability to a "higher" authority (e.g., the CEO, the board of trustees) increases. This lack of self-awareness has led to the career derailments of numerous technically capable and otherwise skilled leaders.

FOSTER POSITIVE ONGOING PERCEPTIONS

Perception does not always equate to reality, but it is what matters most to many employees; it is the equivalent of truth through their organizational lens. Changing a perception once it is widely held is a time-consuming and difficult task for the executive. Likewise, managing and fostering positive perceptions involves a great deal of convincing of staff through honest actions and words, and with careful thought devoted to planning each interaction.

The best first step in managing perception, as it is in managing any task, is to follow the appropriate protocol. Steps in the protocol are enumerated in Exhibit 1.3 and described in detail in the sections that follow. Although general in nature, the protocol provides excellent guidelines for daily behavior as a healthcare executive, and it can serve to foster positive perceptions among staff, peers, and supervisors.

EXHIBIT 1.3: Protocol for Executive Behavior

1. Demonstrate respect for others at all times.
2. Seek constant and diverse feedback.
3. Practice effective communication.
4. Model desired behavior.

Demonstrate Respect for Others at All Times

As many executives move up in their organizations, they may develop a tendency, without realizing it, to grow less tolerant of others' views and backgrounds, thus showing less respect. Their leadership style focuses on implementing their own desires and catering to senior leaders and board members rather than on demonstrating respect to those with whom they interact on a daily basis. To avoid negative perceptions, executives need to be mindful of two key aspects of respect that should guide their actions:

- *Listening.* One of the most effective ways to demonstrate respect for others is to truly listen to them. When employees raise an issue, executives too often fall into the habit of solving the problem based on their experience, rather than allowing the employees to be truly "heard." In these instances, the executives are not listening, but rather waiting for their turn to speak. Effective executives demonstrate the ability to actively listen with understanding and empathy.
- *Common courtesy.* A comparison of executives' behavior around board members and key physicians with their behavior around frontline staff is often telling of how much these executives value certain groups of people. The

true test of leadership character is how a leader treats a person who cannot do anything to advance that leader's career. Staff will quickly pick up on behavior that is condescending or disingenuous.

Seek Constant and Diverse Feedback

The extent to which leaders can reach their full potential within an organization is largely determined by the perception of them by the people whom they have been invited to lead. Healthcare executives, particularly at senior levels, often lack the self-awareness to recognize behaviors that may lead to negative perceptions. They feel that their current behavior has led to their success and that their career advancement has reinforced their personal views. Thus, the open exchange of ideas becomes obsolete from their leadership style.

To avoid the isolation of thought that derails the careers of many senior executives, leaders at all levels should develop mechanisms, both formal and informal, for obtaining regular feedback about their personal leadership performance. Once obtained, this information should be incorporated into the leaders' own professional development plans so that they can constantly evolve their personal leadership skill sets based on the feedback of others. Participating in formal 360-degree evaluations on a regular basis, seeking feedback in standing one-on-one meetings with staff, and encouraging (and respecting) diverse viewpoints in executive team meetings can all help foster frank and honest dialogue that leads to professional growth. Executives should have diversity of thought in mind as they build their teams, and they should understand that the strongest teams, whether in sports or management, are composed of members who have different strengths and viewpoints and who play different roles.

Finally, executives must display the appropriate internal strength of character to create a safe environment for open dialogue and to accept constructive feedback as a gift rather than a criticism. If an executive speaks about seeking feedback but then retaliates against those who provide it, trust will be lost. The result will be a culture of yes-people who seldom give their full opinions and may hide critical facts that might cause their supervisor personal or professional discomfort.

Practice Effective Communication

Executives usually live very busy lives, always running from one commitment to the next. As leaders advance in rank and responsibility, they typically have less time to focus on face-to-face interaction with employees, potentially leading to perceptions of inattentiveness among the rank and file. Department supervisors spend much more time with their staff than do executives; in fact, many frontline leaders spend a majority of their day in the departments they supervise. Because executives have other demands on their time, they must spend it wisely and make up in quality of time what they cannot afford in quantity.

Because they only have a few moments to make a favorable impression, executives should view each of their interactions with employees the way politicians view sound bites during a political campaign. The sound-bite concept applies not only when talking with employees but also when interacting with members of the community. Because executives are the most visible representation of the organization, their statements in social situations are often interpreted as the organization's official stance. Therefore, care should be taken ahead of time to craft specific sound bites that can be used in a variety of situations. The following suggestions can improve the quality of an executive's sound bites:

- *Know and recall key facts.* Be able to speak to the high points of your strategy and the current performance of your organization or department in a clear and concise manner. If you are going into a particular unit of the hospital, speak to the department leader ahead of time to understand the pressing issues or significant staff achievements, and then work them into your sound bites.

- *Be careful with casual comments.* Executives should carefully calculate the impact of comments they make to employees during brief encounters. These fleeting comments can linger and are often repeated to other staff members long after the encounter has passed. Stick as much as you can to your key talking points, and always have a well-prepared general or work-related discussion topic in mind to be used as "filler" if needed.

- *Consider carefully what you say in meetings.* Every sentence or phrase is crucial and can be subject to misinterpretation if repeated out of context. Consider the caution that politicians exercise in polishing every aspect of campaign speeches: Preparation is key to success.

Model Desired Behavior

The behavior of leaders should mirror the stated values of their organizations, and it should be consistent with what the leaders expect of those who work with and for them. For instance, if a leader publicly endorses the values of servant leadership and empowerment but actually practices a strict, top-down, hierarchical approach to management that stifles others' feedback, employees will quickly pick up on the disconnect, and they will begin to see that leader as disingenuous. In leadership, as in life, it is important to practice what you preach.

SUMMARY

A positive perception is something that is earned, and it cannot be granted to leaders by virtue of the titles they hold in their organizations. It is also incredibly fragile. Employee sentiment can shift rapidly if executives do not constantly work to proactively build favorable organizational identities and quickly address any misperceptions the staff may develop. The protocols presented in this chapter provide a framework that can help leaders at all levels. But ultimately, only through honest and consistent effort and genuine behavior can executives gain and hold the trust of those they have been invited to lead.

As you conclude this chapter, focus on these thoughts:

1. It is critical that you develop mechanisms to determine how others perceive you.

2. Leadership is probably not a "50-50" proposition; you need to go the extra step with those who follow you. As in a healthy marriage relationship, perhaps leaders need to go more than halfway.

3. Consider this: People early in their careers typically receive ample feedback on how they are perceived. Those later in their careers usually do not have this type of feedback provided.

GUEST COMMENTARY: SCOTT A. MALANEY

Starting in the mid-1960s, Dr. Gene Jennings wrote extensively about failed executives. After interviewing and studying countless smart, promising people who ultimately failed, he espoused a mind-set he referred to as "other worldliness." This mind-set centered on the idea that success

(continued)

(continued from previous page)

(or failure) at the top is often based on the leader's ability to place himself into the shoes of the other person. To do so is a challenging task. People frequently, if not always, evaluate their own personal behavior based on intent and other people's behavior based on what they did or said. That gap, which is poorly understood, is a danger zone. The leader must seek to reduce the gap between "reality and rhetoric."

The key to understanding the gap, and reducing it, is gathering reliable insight into behavior. In our organization, I am evaluated by many people. All board members, all direct reports, and the entire medical staff are invited to respond to a set of questions to identify how well I am engendering associate and physician support. A wonderful book by Patrick Lencioni, *The Five Dysfunctions of a Team*, reminds us that the most important relationships we have at work are with the other senior leaders. In our organization, we call our senior management group the Executive Steering Council. I am surrounded with people I can trust to provide me the truth, even when it is uncomfortable, and vice versa. We can help reduce the "reality and rhetoric" gap for one another when committed to our collective success.

Maintaining visibility, communicating effectively, and behaving consistently are all key skills of successful leaders. The ability to put yourself in the other person's shoes and then behave accordingly is essential. Having teammates who make sure you receive appropriate real-time feedback about your daily behavior can help make all team members and the organization successful over the long term.

Scott A. Malaney
President and CEO, Blanchard Valley Health System
Findlay, Ohio

REFLECTIVE QUESTIONS

1. You have recently been hired as the CEO of a community hospital, and you are holding your first series of town hall meetings. During a morning session, a nurse stands up and tells you about an article she recently read outlining how CEO pay has risen 10 times faster than average worker wages since 1970. She is concerned about your compensation level because the hospital has fallen on hard times. How would you use the protocols in this chapter to respond to her concerns?

2. You have just been promoted to a manager role in your organization, and you begin to notice that the staff members who were formerly your peers but now report to you are less open with you in terms of issues going on in the organization. What protocol would you employ to make sure you get appropriate feedback about your performance and priorities as you transition into your new role?

RESOURCES AND EXERCISES FOR LEADERSHIP DEVELOPMENT

1. Review the literature on "managerial derailment." Excellent resources include the following:

    Braddy, P. W., J. Gooty, J. W. Fleenor, and F. J. Yammarino. 2014. "Leader Behaviors and Career Derailment Potential: A Multi-analytic Method Examination of Rating Source and Self–Other Agreement." *Leadership Quarterly* 25 (2): 373–90.

    McCartney, W. W., and C. R. Campbell. 2006. "Leadership, Management, and Derailment: A Model of Individual Success and Failure." *Leadership & Organization Development Journal* 27 (3): 190–202.

2. Become intimately familiar with the concept of emotional intelligence.

3. Review the scholarly literature on self-awareness.

4. Review the two chapters on the leadership competencies associated with developing a well-cultivated self-awareness in Dye and Garman's *Exceptional Leadership: 16 Critical Competencies for Healthcare Executives*, second edition (Chicago: Health Administration Press, 2015).

REFERENCES

Gomstyn, A. 2010. "Walmart CEO Pay: More in an Hour Than Workers Get All Year?" *ABC News*. Published July 2. http://abc-news.go.com/Business/walmart-ceo-pay-hours-workers-year/story?id=11067470#.

Lombardo, M. M., and R. W. Eichinger. 2003. *The Leadership Architect Norms and Validity Report*. Minneapolis, MN: Lominger.

————. 2002. *The Leadership Machine: Architecture to Develop Leaders for Any Future*. Minneapolis, MN: Lominger.

Securities and Exchange Commission. 2015. "SEC Adopts Rule for Pay Ratio Disclosure." Published August 5. www.sec.gov/news/pressrelease/2015-160.html.

CHAPTER 2

Professional Image

Envisioning success creates an inspiring image,
but bringing that image to life requires action.

—Larina Kase

Guide to Reader

This chapter continues the discussion that began in the first chapter regarding the importance of perception. Effective leaders take into consideration their professional image. They understand how their image plays a role in their persuasive successes and their ability to interact with all levels and types of people, and also how their demeanor reflects a sense of the appropriate. More than just dress and deportment, professional image incorporates all aspects of what is referred to as "executive presence"; it includes such factors as body language, personality, style of speech, diction, and clarity of communication.

The Importance of Image

The director of a major nursing unit in a well-respected community hospital was the type of leader every executive would want as a member of the management team. She was well prepared academically, had significant experience, achieved exceptional results, and was well liked and respected by staff and physicians alike. For years she had been named on a number of lists for executive-level succession planning, yet she had never been promoted. Although she managed her unit well and had a demonstrated track record of success, her appearance was always a bit disheveled, and her posture was slouched. She contributed positively in group settings, but she often arrived to meetings a few minutes late and appeared to be harried and disorganized. When she was given the opportunity to present her unit's quality plan to the hospital's executive team, she impressed the group with her content knowledge and passion, but her body language was not professional. She tended to ramble as she read from her slides, and she deferred to members of the leadership team during the question and answer session. She also was obviously not comfortable interjecting her thoughts when the factors related to poor performance on key quality metrics were being debated among the executives. As much as the hospital's senior executives liked and respected this talented clinical leader, they never felt quite comfortable moving her to the next level.

Be mindful: Whether in terms of dress, deportment, the way you sit or stand, or the intonation of your voice, the ability to have a "presence" is often a key characteristic of effective leadership. Learning what presence is and how to pull it off is vital. (If you do not manage your image, someone else will.)

WHAT IS A PROFESSIONAL IMAGE?

Image is an interpretation of a persona that is perceived, whether accurately or inaccurately, as the truth. Leaders are constantly under scrutiny, both overtly and covertly, from their audiences. For healthcare executives, these audiences include employees at all levels, whether or not they work directly under the executives; supervisors and middle managers; executive peers; patients; physicians; vendors; and the greater community. Leaders must build and project a positive image in order to lessen, and ideally ward off, negative perceptions from any of these groups. A strong professional image signals the executive's fit within the organization; its effectiveness can be measured by what is real (tangible results) as well as by what seems real (perception).

We have all witnessed leaders who seem to "command the room" and garner instant respect wherever they go. However, the formal definition of a positive professional image, or executive presence, remains elusive. In an era in which healthcare leaders come in a variety of sizes, shapes, and colors, are there common factors that can be groomed in people to help establish positive professional images? A survey of nearly 600 human resources professionals aimed to answer this question by identifying the traits and behaviors that hiring managers most often associated with "executive presence" (Dagley 2013). The results are detailed in Exhibit 2.1.

Some of the traits commonly linked to favorable image were those that seemed to drive early impressions, such as physical characteristics and demeanor. Others, such as values in action and use of power, required the careful evaluation of leadership behaviors over time. Thus, the results suggest that to establish and maintain positive professional images, leaders must focus their energy in two distinct areas:

1. Presenting themselves professionally in appearance
2. Demonstrating actions that align with what the members of organizations expect from their leaders

EXHIBIT 2.1: Characteristics That Contribute to Positive Leadership Image

Characteristic	Number of Comments	% of Comments	Brief Description
Values-in-action	129	22%	Courage, integrity, lack of "ego"
Interpersonal behavior patterns	99	17%	Genuineness, respect, valuing of others
Demeanor	80	14%	Confident, composed, authoritative
Communications	55	9%	Articulate, vocal quality, making oneself heard
Intellect and expertise	54	9%	Analytical skill, vision, domain knowledge
Interpersonal skills	52	9%	Connects easily with people
Outcome delivery ability	38	6%	Energy, takes responsibility, achieves outcomes
Status and reputation	35	6%	Role, networks, achievements, reputation
Physical characteristics	31	5%	Grooming and dress, stature, mannerisms
Power use	16	3%	Extent the person uses fear and enforcement
	589	100%	

Source: Dagley (2013).

HOW IS A POSITIVE PROFESSIONAL IMAGE BUILT?

The time and energy associated with developing specific image traits can vary significantly. However, the protocol shown in Exhibit 2.2

and discussed in the sections that follow provides guidance for leaders at all levels as they seek to enhance their executive image.

EXHIBIT 2.2: Protocol for Enhancing Professional Image

To develop and maintain a positive professional image, leaders should focus on the following key areas:

1. Maintaining professional style
2. Displaying the appropriate demeanor
3. Demonstrating strength of character

Maintaining Professional Style

The manner in which you present yourself can have a tremendous influence on whether the people around you will perceive you as a leader. Style of dress, grooming, mannerisms, and interpersonal behavior must be congruent with what people expect of you and your role in the organization. If people perceive dissonance between a leader's style and the established expectations, that leader's underlying substance and capabilities might be overlooked purely as a result of superficial observations.

In a diverse workforce that usually includes members of four generations, appropriate style is subject to many interpretations. However, a few basic tenets can help to create an image that will be well received in any work situation.

- *Wear appropriate clothing.* In many respects, appropriate executive dress is a uniform dictated by generally accepted professional standards. These standards vary, however, according to regional or cultural practices, so discretion is paramount. Understanding the cultural norms of your own organization is also critical. If the expectation is that executives wear business suits at all times, a director looking to move up the ranks would be wise to dress the part throughout the regular workday. Appropriate executive attire is not intended to express individuality; after all, it is a uniform. Clothes that are too flashy, individualistic, or contemporary are usually inappropriate. A safe measure of whether an outfit is professionally appropriate is to ask others—family, friends, peers—what they would likely notice first, you or your clothes. If the answer is the latter, then the outfit is not for the office.

- *Be careful with business casual.* Business casual or "dress down" days, such as casual Fridays, have made dressing for work even more challenging. Generally, erring on the side of caution when assuming less formal attire is preferred. Many board members, senior executives, and older employees still practice the conservative approach to dressing at work and may not be as accepting of leaders in excessively casual dress. A good rule of thumb: When in doubt, don't.

- *Maintain good hygiene.* This point may seem too basic to even mention in a book geared toward leaders in healthcare, but poor hygiene is nevertheless a factor that can hinder well-qualified, intelligent candidates from advancing in their careers. Bad breath, poor grooming, body odor, and overpowering cologne/perfume are all personal issues that busy leaders might overlook as their schedules become increasingly hectic.

- *Mind personal habits and behavior.* Smoking, chewing gum, talking with your mouth full, and biting your fingernails are just a few of the personal behaviors that some people find offensive. Even seemingly minor bad habits can taint the image of competent leaders and limit their professional success.

- *Maintain a healthy lifestyle.* With healthcare shifting from a focus on acute care to population health management, promoting wellness will be an increasingly important executive competency for industry leaders going forward. Leaders within healthcare will be expected by both employees and the public to model the healthy lifestyle they are promoting for the markets they serve. Following sensible eating habits, maintaining a healthy weight, and exercising regularly will all be expectations of a positive professional image.

Not all of us can look as though we just stepped out of a magazine or can seem so polished that we have no bad habits. However, we can at least try to appear "put together" and well behaved every day. Physical appearance and behavior set the stage for all human interactions. What you say and what you wear are not merely the end results of hygiene or vanity, and covering your mouth when you cough is not just polite happenstance—these are the products of your commitment to yourself. Generally, one's first impression dictates the direction of a meeting and its subsequent outcome. Because the career span of an executive is punctuated, and in some cases propelled by, thousands of brief encounters, success can often be dictated by how well one masters the art of good physical appearance and behavior.

Displaying the Appropriate Demeanor

Today's busy, high-pressure careers have relegated common courtesy and social skills to the back seat of many leaders' consciousness. As a result, stress among executives and staff is increasingly high, and people in general are becoming accustomed to rude behavior. But an appropriate leadership demeanor can convey an overall sense of maturity that can foster respect even in difficult situations. This type of demeanor develops from cultivated ways of being. By practicing the following common social graces and skills, the leader can set a strong example of behavior for the organization and gain a tremendous amount of positive relationship equity:

- *Show common courtesy.* One of the best ways to show courtesy is to demonstrate a strong respect for employees at all levels of the organization, especially those in service areas. Departments such as housekeeping and dietary are often neglected in a healthcare organization, but they have a strong link to key metrics, such as patient satisfaction, and are often home to some of the organization's most dedicated and tenured employees.

- *Demonstrate a strong work ethic.* Ultimately, the staff of an organization takes cues as to what is valued through observation of their leaders. Executives should take pride in their work, have a focus on excellence in everything that they do, prioritize and manage time effectively, and model the behavior they hope to see in all those who work in the organization.

- *Project a positive attitude.* Leaders should not complain without proposing a solution. They should learn to take problems in stride, because complaining only agitates the situation and promotes inaction.

- *Avoid excessive informality.* Though leaders should be collegial with those who work with and for them, interactions need to have a professional line that is not crossed. If you go out for a beer every week with a member of your management team, the personal familiarity that has been built can hamper your efforts to hold that individual accountable if the quality of his work begins to slip. The most productive work settings are those that are open but still have some formality and decorum.

- *Use executive manners both inside and outside of the workplace (and both in town and out of town).* Leaders should consider themselves as representatives of their organization at all times, and their behavior is always on public display. Improper behaviors outside the executive suite can quickly produce negative ramifications inside the suite.

- *Communicate well and be liberal with praise.* The most successful leaders find ways to connect with people. They seek out opportunities to interact with their staff; genuinely express warmth, caring, and concern when appropriate; and make a habit of recognizing employees at all levels who make positive contributions to the organization. Leaders should remember the five-to-one rule: In all their staff interactions, they should deliver five messages of praise for every one criticism. Following this rule will help build a tremendous amount of goodwill and relationship equity that can be called upon to drive positive results.

A leader might demonstrate the appropriate professional behavior and make a great first impression, but the leader's *personal* demeanor is often what makes this impression last. Appropriate leadership style can instill a sense of confidence and convince the staff that you are a caring leader attuned to employees' needs. But if executives have style but are devoid of personality, they will quickly be perceived as "empty suits" without substance.

Demonstrating Strength of Character

In ancient times, the word *character* referred to a distinguishing mark or symbol scratched permanently on a surface. In the context of leadership, *character* still refers to a distinguishing mark, but this time the mark is on the person. Character reflects the inner values and personal traits that make up the foundation of the leader as a human being. It is the collection of essential beliefs that drive our behavior, and it reveals the true person we are in the mirror when no one is watching. Character represents the values-in-action response that hiring managers, in the study discussed earlier, identified as the most important aspect of a positive professional image.

Sustained success in an organization can only be achieved through leaders who demonstrate strength of character. In an ideal world, all executives would possess strong character and thus would always behave appropriately—because doing so would be the natural expression of their inner selves. In reality, however, we are all imperfect individuals with strengths and weaknesses of character, and we all must work to enhance our character to improve our conduct and influence. The following behaviors are good exercises for building effective character:

- *Be the same person every day.* Few things are more disconcerting to staff than dealing with a boss who is prone to intense mood swings and erratic behavior. A leader should provide steady guidance with consistency of personality and management style. Such guidance allows staff to shape their thought processes and behavior around predictable expectations.

- *Be honest in all interactions.* Credibility is the most powerful tool that leaders have to drive their organizations to sustained success. It is what enables them to convince others—superiors, peers, and subordinates—to believe in the direction the leaders set and to put in their best efforts to achieve common goals. Trust is the base of all credibility. Trust takes time to establish, but it can be destroyed in an instant if an executive is dishonest. The wrong words, especially untruths, can permanently damage an executive's credibility and may irrevocably harm their ability to lead and influence others. Distortion, withholding facts, and exaggeration are all forms of dishonesty common in healthcare organizations, usually because they ease the burden of difficult decision making by only representing the details people want to hear. In the end, however, the truth typically is revealed, and the concealing of facts does greater damage to relationships than transparency would have.
- *Promise only what can be done.* Leaders should be cautious about promising, or even suggesting, anything unless they are absolutely certain the commitment will come to fruition. If a leader says she will do something, then she must do it or credibility will be lost. Leaders should avoid situations where suggestions might be made but not precisely fulfilled—for instance, discussing promotional opportunities with subordinates that are not yet approved.
- *Personalize difficult decisions.* Executives sometimes make global decisions for their organizations without fully considering the impact on their employees. Layoffs, terminations, and the reduction or elimination of programs must be done occasionally, even in well-run organizations. However, leaders should not finalize these kinds of decisions without first imagining themselves as the recipient of the bad news, rather than the giver. The

human costs involved in decisions or actions are often what ultimately make or break plans and programs.

- *Give, and be willing to receive, forgiveness.* Executives are human and thus, by definition, imperfect individuals. All leaders make mistakes in their careers, but the most successful ones have a habit of correcting those mistakes by delivering gracious apologies and learning from the experiences. Likewise, all the people who work for leaders will also have missteps; the task of a mature leader is to create a safe environment where honest mistakes can be openly discussed and not handled in a punitive manner.

- *Avoid temptation.* History is littered with stories of powerful leaders who fall from grace because of some moral failing. The best way to avoid such mishaps in your career is to avoid placing yourself in potentially compromising situations. Welcome oversight and external auditing of your expense reports, and avoid extremely informal meetings with staff, particularly those of the opposite sex. Be certain to have at least one trusted adviser outside your chain of command who can serve as your sounding board and moral compass if you encounter situations that you fear might border on unethical.

General Norman Schwarzkopf, the leader of the allied forces in the first Gulf War, viewed leadership as character in action. He said, "Leadership is a potent combination of strategy and character. But if you must be without one, be without strategy" (Schwarzkopf and Petre 1992). If leaders fail to approach their roles with strength of character, not even the most polished style or pleasant disposition will save them from losing credibility with their staff over time. In the end, the success or failure of every leader depends on how well he demonstrates his values in daily actions.

Today, an additional part of your professional image is reflected through the use of social media. This important topic deserves its own chapter and is discussed in depth in Chapter 10.

SUMMARY

For executives to be effective in any organization, they must garner and sustain the trust and respect of those who work with and for them. In an image-conscious world, leaders must look the part and pass the scrutiny of an increasingly discerning audience with very specific ideas of how a leader should present and behave. Style in and of itself, however, is not enough to maintain a positive professional image. Over time, leaders are judged more broadly, based on their actions and the content of their characters.

Readers should conclude this chapter with these three thoughts:

1. Often, the "little things," such as eye contact (or lack thereof), body language, dress, and attention to grooming and personal appearance, will make or break you as you seek to lead in your organization. Individual attention to this level of detail can be critical.

2. Yes, your competence and even your character are judged by your looks.

3. Do you know what people say about you when you are not in the room? If you do not, you are missing a valuable piece of information that can propel you to greater success.

GUEST COMMENTARY: J. ERIC EVANS

Most would concede that a positive professional image is critical for career success, but the topic is often addressed only in amorphous terms. Professional image means different things to different people, with interpretations ranging from attire to communication style. Because of its subjective nature, feedback about professional image is often taken personally or readily dismissed. However, whether obtained from your boss, from colleagues, or through self-reflection, professional image feedback provides precious insights that can empower you to shape and control your career success.

In leadership, every decision we make, our approaches to challenging situations, our reactions to failure and success, and even how we spend our free time are closely observed. Each day is an ongoing interview process for our careers. As such, we must recognize that professional image is not formed in a vacuum or only in defining moments such as when we are making important presentations or interacting with superiors. Our daily interactions with all levels of staff, community leaders, and patients/customers are where the foundation of professional image is formed and judged. The constancy of perception formation requires that positive professional image be rooted in core beliefs and genuine intent. Anything less than authentic leadership will become transparent, and trying to be someone you are not is a plan destined to fail.

The good news is that professional image is not dependent on personality traits, fashion sense, or physical stature. People with outstanding executive presence come in all

(continued)

(continued from previous page)

shapes and sizes and have varying leadership styles. In my experience, leaders with a great professional image do the following:

- Compartmentalize their day and remain present and engaged. Regardless of what else is happening or how the previous meeting went, these leaders have the discipline to focus on the task at hand in ways that others rely on and respect.

- Consciously *act*, rather than *react*, regardless of the stakes or context. The ability to constructively navigate conflict, avoid emotional responses, and focus on the end game often has a disproportionate impact on professional image.

- Admit when they don't know something or when they make a mistake. Effective leaders—and the majority of employees—understand that willingness to admit failure or lack of knowledge is not a weakness but rather a sign of strength. Alternatively, the inability to appear fallible often proves to significantly weaken leadership influence and image.

All of these behaviors rarely come to an individual naturally. Developing a positive professional image starts with disciplined self-reflection and openness to feedback, as outlined in this chapter. I will leave you with two tips to consider as part of your continuous improvement toolkit for professional image:

- Make a habit of asking yourself, "How are others experiencing me right now?" throughout your day. I

(continued)

(continued from previous page)

learned this tip from a business school professor, and it never fails to quiet my mind and keep me focused.

- Until that becomes habit, explicitly schedule two or three ten-minute time blocks throughout your day, and use this time to step back and evaluate your interactions and successes thus far and to refocus on the interactions yet to come.

J. Eric Evans
Market Chief Executive Officer
Sierra Providence Health Network
Providence Memorial and Providence Children's Hospital
El Paso, Texas

REFLECTIVE QUESTIONS

1. One of your peer managers aspires to move up in the organization but has not been promoted, despite good work performance. You suspect that his relatively unkempt appearance and overly informal demeanor may be preventing the senior leadership from viewing him as a potential senior manager. How might you thoughtfully approach this topic with him?

2. To what extent might the situation in Question 1 be more difficult if there is a gender difference between you and your peer?

3. Reflect on a supervisor you have had in your career who garnered a great deal of trust and respect across the organization. What attributes of character did this person

display that you might want to emulate to enhance your own professional image?

RESOURCES AND EXERCISES FOR LEADERSHIP DEVELOPMENT

1. Run an Internet search on "personal image consultants" or "executive image consultants" and determine what material might be pertinent to your image development.

2. A significant amount of material relating to professional image correlates to gender. Find a professional friend of the opposite gender with whom you can have a detailed discussion on how gender differences impact professional image.

REFERENCES

Dagley, G. R. 2013. *Executive Presence: Influence Beyond Authority*. Melbourne: Australian Human Resources Institute.

Schwarzkopf, H. N., and P. Petre. 1992. *It Doesn't Take a Hero*. New York: Bantam.

CHAPTER 3

Professional Reputation

You can't build a reputation on what you are going to do.

—Henry Ford

Guide to Reader

Professional reputation differs from the concept of professional image discussed in the previous chapter. In a sense, whereas image is built, reputation is earned. Image connotes a calculated attempt to represent yourself, to establish what is often called your "personal brand"; it has a certain degree of superficiality. Reputation, on the other hand, is based mostly on your results and on the manner in which you achieve those results. It might be said that reputation is more important than image. Within the context of this book, both are important, but reputation, once lost, is much more difficult to regain.

The Best of Intentions

A young executive had spent several years advancing through the ranks of a formal leadership development program in a major investor-owned hospital chain, and he was excited to finally receive a chance to serve in the CEO role at a small community hospital in a rapidly growing suburb. He felt confident that he had the technical skills and knowledge base to effectively manage and grow the facility, and he had developed an excellent reputation within the broader company as a leader who was responsive, communicated well, and produced outstanding results. He also knew that one of the key responsibilities he would have in his new role would be to represent the hospital in the community, which was not something he had done to a great extent during his development program. Recognizing this area as a deficit, he embraced the opportunity wholeheartedly. He began volunteering for board seats at the local chamber of commerce, a couple of charitable organizations, and some social clubs. This involvement quickly led to invitations to social events nearly every evening, as well as frequent luncheons during work hours. The CEO found himself overextended, frequently having to cancel commitments both inside and outside of the organization. As a result, his reputation in the community soon became one of being "too busy" and "unreliable." The competing priorities also caused his work product to slip, ultimately tarnishing his reputation within the company as well. What started as a noble endeavor to become integrated into the community nearly derailed the young executive's career trajectory.

Be mindful: Unlike titles, a professional reputation cannot be given or taken away; it can only be earned over time through your words and actions.

PROFESSIONAL REPUTATION VERSUS PROFESSIONAL IMAGE

If a professional image is the cover of the book that determines how a leader is initially perceived, then a professional reputation represents the pages that make up the story of how the leader is ultimately regarded. A reputation may at first be crafted by the way an executive behaves, but the manner in which the reputation evolves is determined largely by the actions and interpretations of others. In this regard, a professional reputation takes on a very real life of its own, made up of the collective mental construct that other people hold and share about an individual.

To better understand the relationship between professional reputation and professional image, consider the model shown in Exhibit 3.1. First, values, beliefs, and attitudes help shape the executive's personal leadership philosophy. Together, these elements sit "beneath the surface" and provide a foundation for the external behaviors demonstrated by the leader on a daily basis. These behaviors form the visible "tip of the iceberg" that rises from the values, beliefs, and attitudes. The leader's observed behaviors and interactions then aggregate to form the professional reputation. Note that image is more superficial—yet still important—and sits atop both reputation and the values and belief system. Exhibit 3.2 demonstrates how the "iceberg" constructed in Exhibit 3.1 drives personal and organizational results—and also how those results, in turn, affect professional reputation and image.

HOW TO DEVELOP PROFESSIONAL REPUTATION

Over the span of a career, a professional reputation can be a tangible asset and a key differentiating factor in a competitive job market. All executives, therefore, should actively work to cultivate it. They should strive to develop and maintain a positive reputation,

EXHIBIT 3.1: Relationship Between Professional Reputation and Professional Image

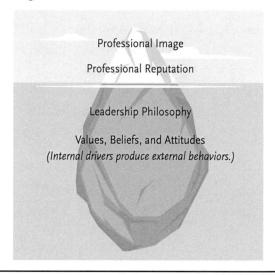

EXHIBIT 3.2: Reputation, Image, and Personal and Organizational Results

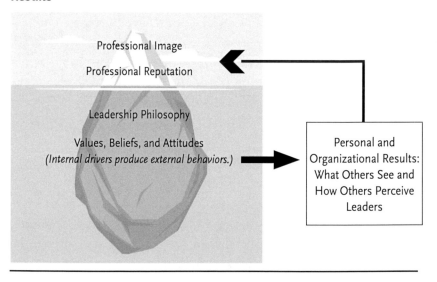

both inside and outside the office, that reflects their personal values and transcends the immediate needs and duties of their careers.

In recent years, many books on leadership have begun referring to reputations as "leadership brands," underscoring the notion that executives should spend the same amount of time and energy on managing their professional reputations that major organizations devote to building and protecting their corporate brands (Schawbel 2009). Because reputation management is not taught in business school, leaders seeking to improve in this area may benefit from the protocol shown in Exhibit 3.3 and described in the sections that follow.

EXHIBIT 3.3: Protocol for Enhancing Professional Reputation

The following steps can guide the development of a positive professional reputation:

1. Understand your current reputation.
2. Define your desired personal brand.
3. Craft your reputational marketing strategy.
4. Implement and update.

Understand Your Current Reputation

Before you can determine how to enhance your professional reputation, you must first establish a baseline understanding of how you are currently perceived. Participate in a 360-degree evaluation; have personal meetings with peers, subordinates, and supervisors to obtain feedback; and have frank conversations with individuals outside of the organization (former employees, community members) about what they perceive to be your strengths and weaknesses. Approach these discussions with a true desire to learn, creating a safe environment for honest feedback, and do not question or take offense to any constructive criticism you receive. At the end of the process, you should garner a good understanding of the opinions others hold of you today.

Define Your Desired Personal Brand

Perhaps the most important thing to remember about reputations is that they are not static. They are constantly evolving, and leaders can seek to define them and influence how they change over time. No single management style or personality type predisposes someone to be considered a great leader, so leaders should individually decide how they would like to be known in their organizations and in the community. As leaders interact with and observe other leaders during the course of their careers, they should develop a mental construct of the behaviors they have witnessed in others that they would hope to emulate.

Leaders will likely have significant variations in their desired personal brands. Some may wish to be known as tough leaders who are able to make effective decisions in difficult situations; others may want their primary brand to be one of being intelligent or approachable. Some may want to be known as "turn-around" leaders. Remember that, although leaders can influence their reputations through intentional activities and communication, they cannot convincingly create and sustain a reputation over time that is contrary to their personal values and beliefs. Simply put, eventually there will be dissonance, and that dissonance will be detected by those with whom the leaders interact. Any desired leadership brand needs to be consistent with the values system of the leader and the organization he serves.

Once a leader has defined her desired professional reputation, she should perform a gap analysis between the desired state and her understanding of her current reputation. This analysis, which relies on a robust feedback system, will identify focus areas that the leader should address to enhance her reputation. Exhibit 3.4 provides a sample action chart to help in this process.

EXHIBIT 3.4: Sample Gap Analysis for Personal Branding Improvement

How I Want to Be Known	How I Am Currently Perceived (Based on Perceptions and Results)	Identified Gaps	Personal Action Plan
High-visibility leader	Lower employee engagement scores; not enough rounding or time out of office		
Person of action	Too many objectives; too demanding		
Leader in patient excellence	Patient satisfaction scores; average patient quality		

Craft Your Reputational Marketing Strategy

Once leaders recognize the distance that exists between their current and desired reputations, they must create plans to close the gaps and build more effective professional brands. Just as companies routinely develop marketing strategies to enhance their brand equity with defined audiences, leaders should have formal strategies to modify their actions, interpersonal relationships, and professional networking. Leaders should not only define the actions they will take to enhance their brand but also identify key audiences they will target as they look to deploy their strategy. If an executive wishes to be known as a visible and open leader but has received feedback that the frontline staff feel disconnected from him, then his personal reputational marketing strategy should include more opportunities for positive interactions with rank-and-file employees.

Leaders must recognize that their reputations need to be groomed both inside and outside their organizations; however, balancing internal and external pursuits can be a challenge. Our opening chapter vignette illustrates vividly that executives who become too preoccupied with external activities run the risk of neglecting internal responsibilities and ultimately hurting their organizations' performance. Nonetheless, executives must effectively represent their organizations in their communities and participate in professional organizations that foster continued growth. The internal and external aspects of a leader's responsibility will continually compete for time, and the key to maintaining a positive reputation is to strike an effective balance.

Building an Effective Reputation Outside the Organization

Building a reputation among one's peers outside the organization requires active participation in local and national professional and trade organizations. These organizations, such as the American College of Healthcare Executives (ACHE), provide a forum in which careerists in similar professions can network, pursue continuing education and professional development, and set standards of behavior by which all members are expected to abide. The organizations also afford executives the opportunity to contribute to the professional body of knowledge by sharing best practices, publishing, and teaching courses and seminars—all of which can help build a positive reputation within the industry.

Remember also that healthcare leaders do not develop their professional reputations strictly within the field of healthcare. Therefore, participation in community organizations such as the local chamber of commerce and service clubs such as Rotary is another key to success.

Because most healthcare organizations depend significantly on government-sponsored healthcare payers—and because the Affordable Care Act in 2010 brought fundamental changes to the healthcare field—leaders must become versed in public advocacy. Executives can enhance their professional reputations by providing legislative input and participating actively in professional organizations that lobby to protect the interests of healthcare delivery systems, such as the American Hospital Association (AHA).

Building an Effective Reputation Inside the Organization

Leaders build their reputations within the organizations they lead through the behaviors they exhibit every day. With each interaction, staff will form a mental construct of what they think of their leaders and of how they will verbally portray those leaders to others. Employees in a healthcare setting expect their leaders to provide a vision and set goals for the organization, to have an infectious positive attitude about where the organization is going, to be engaged and visible, to express empathy and caring, to recognize staff for their contributions, and to place the patient at the center of all decisions. Executives should craft their desired leadership brands with these expectations in mind, and they should focus on building these competencies while remaining genuine to their own personal values.

Implement and Update

Once leaders have developed an understanding of the types of reputations they would like to build and have crafted formal plans of development, they should implement their strategies with the same fervor of a major brand advertising campaign. As with any behavioral change, it may take some time for target audiences to recognize the efforts being put forward.

Consistency of behavior is crucial, and leaders should use all tools available—body language, interpersonal communication, public forums, and even social media—to reinforce their images. Leaders cannot sit back and hope that their actions are being noticed; instead, they must intentionally build networks through all interactions. Over time, a professional reputation will be created. As leaders deploy their personal branding strategies, they should use a close network of coaches (i.e., trusted confidants and mentors) who can provide honest and useful critiques.

Become a Thought Leader

Contrary to popular wisdom, a thought leader is not necessarily an individual who always develops brand-new, innovative ideas. Thought leaders are often those individuals who stay current on new trends and adapt aspects of those trends for their organizations. Dye and Garman (2015) write that these individuals often are able to "synthesize people's ideas into a coherent whole" and "recognize common themes and trends, and effectively articulate them."

SUMMARY

Leadership is largely based on effective interactions with others. When you lead, your decisions will not be universally applauded. Each interpersonal interaction introduces risk to you. You might rub someone the wrong way, you might create an improper impression, or you might have difficulty getting through to some people. You can't always stop others from questioning your judgment or speaking ill of you, but a positive reputation affords you the benefit of the doubt in many such instances. Members of your network might rise to your defense, oftentimes without you even knowing about it. A positive professional brand can make you a role model, providing a motivational stimulus that inspires others and sets a standard for younger members of the profession.

A good reputation is fragile, needs constant cultivation, and is much more difficult to build than to destroy. Nurturing a positive reputation requires consistent and purposeful effort, patience, and time; yet that reputation can crumble with a single misstep. All healthcare leaders should make it a priority to effectively manage their professional brand. Remember that the best way to maintain a good reputation is to become a person who deserves one.

As you conclude this chapter, focus on these four thoughts:

1. With the trappings of power, authority, and status and the benefits that come with higher-level leadership positions, leaders often lose their grounding and do not stay centered.

2. For this chapter and many others in this book, a profound understanding of the concept of managerial derailment may help leaders retain their ability to see "true north."

3. The higher up leaders move in organizations, the less likely they are to receive unfettered feedback on issues of reputation.

4. A professional reputation is the most important asset in your career; guard it accordingly.

GUEST COMMENTARY: BRITT T. REYNOLDS

I have been afforded, over my 27-year career, influence and direction from three key mentors, and each of these role models has espoused and demonstrated the value of honesty and integrity at the core of leadership. A reputation built on honesty and integrity, in all interactions, is paramount. This grounding must be uncompromised regardless of situational challenges or circumstances; yet this foundation also allows for leadership adaptability and flexibility.

(continued)

(continued from previous page)

This foundation, when coupled with the discipline of self-reflection, enhances intrinsic awareness as well as interpersonal relationships. It leads to healthy curiosity and honest self-assessment, which help shape reputation as well as brand image. Self-assessment and feedback from others develop and strengthen a leader's character. This strength of character allows for equal embracing of limitations and celebration of successes. Once individuals are comfortable with a leader's character, a safety for feedback results. A healthy environment is reflected in such processes as 360-degree assessments and formal mentorship.

A fundamental element of building and maintaining one's reputation is transparency. The transparency born from a foundation of honesty and integrity manifests as "genuineness" in others' interpretations. When a leader's reputation includes genuineness, the leader creates an open invitation for critique and develops effectiveness in self-improvement. Additionally, transparency helps foster clear and effective communication, another virtue critical to a solid reputation.

To achieve desired results, an ideal end state, reputation is brokered and communication is key. When communication is honest, transparent, clear, and direct, reputation is enhanced. I have found that the ability to effectively communicate "why" in all interactions is critical. By challenging leaders to consistently communicate "why," regardless of topic and magnitude, and to consistently hear the "why," accountability can be naturally created and

(continued)

(continued from previous page)

engagement enhanced. Such steps are essential for driving results, which are at the core of one's reputation.

The blending of these elements—a foundation of honesty and integrity, the discipline of self-awareness and curiosity, the methodical pursuit of transparent feedback, and the rigor of clearly and consistently communicating "why"—is paramount to building a strong reputation. Once these elements have been combined, the most important action a leader must take is to identify and engage a colleague to serve as a reputation accountability partner. Such a relationship will ensure grounding, modification when necessary, objective assessment, mutual investment in one another's success, and, most important, a healthy means to grow, develop, refine, and protect one's professional reputation.

Britt T. Reynolds
President, Hospital Operations
Tenet Healthcare
Dallas, Texas

REFLECTIVE QUESTIONS

1. You just celebrated your first 90 days in a new leadership role, and you took part in a 360-degree evaluation of your performance to date. You are surprised to read in the feedback that your staff considers you a bit of an autocratic leader who does not actively seek their input. This assessment is in direct opposition to the way you view your own leadership style. How would you begin to build a different reputation within the organization?

2. Take a moment to reflect on your personal leadership style and the leadership reputation you would like to build. Walk through the protocol in this chapter to define your desired leadership brand and to identify specific actions you will implement to begin shaping your professional reputation.

3. We like this quote from Socrates: "Regard your good name as the richest jewel you can possibly be possessed of—for credit is like fire; when once you have kindled it you may easily preserve it, but if you once extinguish it, you will find it an arduous task to rekindle it again. The way to gain a good reputation is to endeavor to be what you desire to appear." Exactly what do you do to ensure that you practice behavior that supports a "good name"? List those actions on paper.

RESOURCES AND EXERCISES FOR LEADERSHIP DEVELOPMENT

1. Meet with your elected American College of Healthcare Executives (ACHE) Regent and ask how you might help in ACHE chapter activities or other ACHE matters.

2. Consider opportunities to support educational opportunities in your ACHE local chapter.

3. If you are more advanced in your career, consider ways to mentor others.

REFERENCES

Dye, C. F., and A. N. Garman. 2015. *Exceptional Leadership: 16 Critical Competencies for Healthcare Executives*, 2nd ed. Chicago: Health Administration Press.

Schawbel, D. 2009. *Me 2.0: Build a Powerful Brand to Achieve Career Success.* New York: Kaplan.

CHAPTER 4

Ethical Decision Making

There is no right way to do the wrong thing.

—Ken Blanchard

Guide to Reader

Enron, Arthur Andersen, HealthSouth. Readers are urged to give particular thought to this chapter and ensure that they put these principles and guidelines to work at all times. Too often, leaders engage in "ethical relativism" in situations that may not seem to have clear-cut right or wrong answers. Readers should also be aware of the danger of gradual lapses in ethical behavior.

A Slippery Slope

A once-thriving community hospital had fallen on hard times recently, and the CEO was frantically working on a plan to improve the organization's financial performance. Her facility was in a "first ring" suburb of a major metropolitan area, and the demographics of the service area's population had shifted significantly in recent years. Several major businesses had moved their regional offices to a neighboring community, and the population growth and development of new homes had followed those well-paying jobs. A competing healthcare system had been proactive in establishing a strong presence in the fast-growing area, and the CEO of the once-thriving hospital saw a significant deterioration of volumes and payer mix as the out-migration of young insured families continued.

The hospital was owned by a healthcare management company that set aggressive annual goals around volume and revenue growth for all its facilities, and a large percentage of the CEO's income (and job security) was predicated on meeting these goals. She had been falling under increasing pressure for the hospital's declining performance, and her supervisor had recently told her that she had six months to reverse the negative volume trends before the company might have to make a change in leadership.

In reviewing the key volume trends, the CEO noticed that the largest drop in inpatient volume was attributable to fewer admissions coming through the Emergency Department. She discussed this matter with the administrative and medical directors responsible for

(continued)

(continued from previous page)

emergency services to identify the key factors contributing to the decline. She learned that, although the overall number of patients arriving to the Emergency Department was actually growing, the patients were frequently of lower acuity, which resulted in fewer admissions on a percentage basis. Desperately seeking any solution to her volume crisis, the CEO began meeting daily with the Emergency Department medical staff, questioning the physicians' decisions, and demanding that a specific percentage of patients be admitted to the hospital, even if the admission criteria had to be very liberally applied.

These steps produced a short-term increase in volumes for the hospital, but they infuriated the staff. The doctors felt they had been put in a position of having to make what they considered unethical decisions to admit patients who did not need to be in the hospital. After a few months, insurance companies began to retrospectively deny a number of the inpatient claims because many patients did not meet inpatient admission criteria. The physicians reached out to the hospital's management company and the local press to complain that they were being placed in a position of driving inpatient volume against their better judgment. After an investigation, the CEO was fired for unethical leadership and for exposing the company to potentially damaging legal and financial consequences.

Be mindful: Leaders are judged not only on the decisions they make but also on the manner in which they make those decisions. Difficult choices are inevitably a part of any leadership role, so leaders at all levels must consistently apply a mental framework and set of values that can help them navigate these dilemmas in a fair and ethical manner.

THE IMPORTANCE OF ETHICS

Corporate scandals have become so common and well documented in recent decades that the public has seemingly become desensitized to the idea of corrupt executives. From the Enron accounting fiasco that left thousands out of work and without a retirement fund to the BP oil spill caused by corporate leaders who ignored safety codes for the sake of increased financial returns, concerns about ethics in leadership have appeared in news headlines with an increasing frequency. What would drive well-trained and highly capable business leaders to such significant lapses in judgment?

In his best-selling book *Complications,* Harvard-trained surgeon Dr. Atul Gawande (2003) chronicles the process by which talented and well-meaning physicians become "problem" doctors with track records of questionable clinical and ethical decision making. He suggests that these men and women are not evil by any means. Instead, he found during discussions with the physicians that their bad patterns of behavior started very gradually, often without them noticing. Then the behavior accelerated until there was no hope of recovery. Gawande also found that external pressures were often contributing factors in the doctors' behavior change. For example, decreasing reimbursement for surgical cases could cause an already busy surgeon to take on more cases to meet personal financial obligations. To accommodate these additional cases, the surgeon might "cut corners" in terms of quality or surgical technique, or work long hours to the point of becoming unsafe. By the time the physician realizes that the increased workload cannot be maintained, the small steps toward unethical behavior have already spiraled out of control.

Lapses of ethical judgment by business leaders occur in a similar fashion. Most executives, particularly in healthcare, chose their professions because of a legitimate desire to help others. However, external factors, such as changing regulations or pressure to meet financial goals, can threaten to move even the most ethical leaders on a perilous pathway toward unethical decisions. The initial ethical concessions might be diminutive, such as "fudging" an expense report, but they often start a trend toward increasingly egregious behavior that can end in ruin.

The importance of ethics in leadership is heightened in healthcare. The privilege of leading those who care for our neighbors is a sacred trust, and this trust must be actively earned each day. Evidence has shown that corporations with strong ethical reputations not only perform better in staff and customer satisfaction surveys but also demonstrate more favorable financial returns. Executives who wish to create sustained competitive advantage for their organizations conduct themselves as though someone is watching them at all times. The belief that one can get away with unethical behavior because minor lapses in judgment may go unnoticed underestimates the scrutiny placed on leaders of modern organizations.

ENHANCING ETHICAL DECISION MAKING

Effective leaders should begin with a deep commitment to ethical behavior. The internal "compass" serves as a guide and helps resist temptation. When possible, leaders should also develop organizational standards for ethical behavior. The written codification of acceptable behavior provides visible reminders of the established rules and standards. The following protocol, summarized in Exhibit 4.1, aims to assist executives in leading ethically.

EXHIBIT 4.1: Protocol for Ethical Leadership

Leaders should consider the following steps to enhance ethical decision making:

1. Develop a deep personal commitment to ethical behavior.
2. Create and follow an organizational code of ethics.
3. Adhere to a professional code of ethics.
4. Maintain personal ethical standards.

Develop a Deep Personal Commitment to Ethical Behavior

Ethics begins with a personal commitment and a feeling about what is the right thing to do. It is based on morality, justice, and a desire to avoid hurting others. It also involves being comfortable with one's actions if they were to be seen by the public eye.

In assessing the ethics of a particular action, consider the following five questions:

1. Is it right? (based on absolute principles of morality)
2. Is it fair? (based on principles of justice)
3. Who gets hurt? (the fewer, the better)
4. Would you be comfortable if the details of your actions were made public?
5. What would you tell your child, sibling, or young relative to do?

Create and Follow an Organizational Code of Ethics

The organizational code of ethics should be board developed and board driven. It can be authored by the CEO, but the board must support and openly endorse it. Ideally, the code of ethics should be displayed clearly so the entire organization is aware of it. The mission statement of the organization may also reference ethical behavior. The organization should publish policies on regulatory compliance, fiduciary responsibility, and conflicts of interest. The policies should describe specific behavioral expectations that cannot be ignored. The behaviors should become the basis for hiring protocols, reward and recognition programs, and performance reviews, and they should be enforced with progressive discipline when needed.

Adhere to a Professional Code of Ethics

Every profession has a code of ethics, whether published or tacit. However, these codes are only as good as the sanctions used to enforce them and the willingness of professionals to subscribe to the codes and to police themselves. All leaders in healthcare should become familiar with the professional *Code of Ethics* of the American College of Healthcare Executives (ACHE). This comprehensive code, published at www.ache.org/abt_ache/code.cfm, suggests guidelines for behavior, addresses ethical dilemmas commonly faced by leaders in healthcare, and advises leaders in appropriate conduct. It can also be a good source of reference material to help establish or update organizational and personal codes of ethics.

Maintain Personal Ethical Standards

Ethical situations demand consistent responses over time, and ethical leaders thrive through their consistency of behavior. Leaders should establish a personal code of ethics that they hold sacrosanct. For every decision, serious consideration should be given to ethical implications, and the end goal should be for the greater good of the organization and the patients it serves.

SUMMARY

The ultimate cause of unethical behavior is selfishness, and transgressions are often motivated by thoughts of personal gain. Healthcare is, by definition, a service industry, and those who are invited to lead healthcare organizations should do so understanding that their career is one of service to others. Leaders should conduct themselves accordingly and always consider themselves to be under scrutiny. An executive's reputation and credibility are constantly subject to challenge, so ethical behavior should be considered in the context of absolutes. Although answers in management are not always easy or clear-cut, there is no "grading on a curve" when it comes to dealing with ethical imperatives. Simply put, when in doubt, do not do it.

GUEST COMMENTARY: JOE THOMASON

Doing the "right thing" in each and every situation is sometimes difficult but always essential. I had a conversation with a life-long friend who had recently purchased a large manufacturing company. He and I spoke about the challenges and successes he has had with the newly acquired company, including one employee incident that prompted him to put principle over profit.

(continued)

(continued from previous page)

A long-tenured and high-revenue-producing salesperson had revealed to my friend that he had been involved in a personal situation that was illegal, causing my friend to consult the officers of the company and of course the human resource leadership. My friend explained, "I really believed that the individual was remorseful and did retain a large degree of company history and relationships. However, I couldn't get over the personal facts of the situation and didn't know if trust could be reestablished. And most important, he violated the law. We terminated his employment the next day." Affirmation of a decision well made came in the following days with a call from the company's largest client, who assured my friend that he would continue his business relationship with the company.

In the healthcare setting, ethical decision making must impact every aspect of the care provided. Positive outcomes for our patients depend on such decisions. In fact, every time patients enter our facilities, they are expressing their belief that we will do the "right thing" 100 percent of the time. To meet this standard, we must recognize that healthcare is a highly complex and heavily regulated field with many moving parts—including frequent changes to our laws. It is essential for healthcare leaders to stay abreast of this ever-changing environment, model ethical decision making, and accept nothing less in the organizations they lead.

Joe Thomason
Chief Executive Officer
Centennial Medical Center
Frisco, Texas

REFLECTIVE QUESTIONS

1. Consider the case described in the vignette at the beginning of this chapter. What were some of the personal and environmental factors that led this executive to make an unethical decision? How could they have been avoided?

2. Does your organization have a formal code of ethics? If so, find a copy and read it, and then compare the behavior you observe in the organization with what is stated in the code. Is there a disconnect? If so, how might the organization go about addressing it?

RESOURCES AND EXERCISES FOR LEADERSHIP DEVELOPMENT

1. Review the American College of Healthcare Executives (ACHE) *Code of Ethics* (www.ache.org/abt_ache/code.cfm) and the section of the ACHE website that offers suggestions on how to use it (www.ache.org/abt_ache/EthicsToolkit /UsingCode.cfm). Consider using the ACHE *Code* for a discussion group with some of your peer leaders.

2. In addition to the *Code*, ACHE also provides an ethics self-assessment (www.ache.org/newclub/career/ethself.cfm). Take the assessment and consider your responses.

3. Review the following articles:

   Rolland, P. 2008. "Whistle Blowing in Healthcare: An Organizational Failure in Ethics and Leadership." *Internet Journal of Law, Healthcare and Ethics* 6 (1). http://ispub.com/IJLHE/6/1/9204.

   Silva, M. C. 1998. "Organizational and Administrative Ethics in Health Care: An Ethics Gap." *Online Journal*

of Issues in Nursing 3 (3). www.nursingworld.org
/MainMenuCategories/ANAMarketplace/ANA
Periodicals/OJIN/TableofContents/Vol31998
/No3Dec1998/EthicsGap.aspx.

4. Study the ethical guidelines published on the website of the
National Association for Healthcare Quality (www.nahq.org
/Quality-Community/content/codeethicspractice.html).

5. Though this chapter dealt primarily with ethics from a
leadership or executive perspective, many other aspects
of patient care and quality also have ethical dimensions.
If possible, consider serving on your organization's ethics
committee or institutional review board (IRB).

REFERENCE

Gawande, A. 2003. *Complications.* New York: Picador.

CHAPTER 5

Interpersonal Relationships

You do not lead people by hitting them over the head—
that's assault, not leadership.

—Dwight D. Eisenhower

Guide to Reader

Some leaders contend that interpersonal relationships
are the most important requirement for highly effective
leadership. In the words of one CEO, "At the end of the day,
it is how you get along with others that counts the most."
Knowing how others perceive them is often the most
challenging task for leaders, and the challenge presents
itself regardless of the level in the organization at which the
leaders sit.

Great Expectations

A new department manager had recently been promoted because of his strong work ethic and uncanny ability to "get things done." Though he continued his track record of achieving results, early into his tenure he also started to leave bodies in his wake. In less than a year, his entire supervisory team had turned over through a combination of firings and resignations. Worse yet, none of his staff within the department asked to be considered for the open positions, even though the positions represented promotional opportunities and more compensation.

During the exit interviews with the departing supervisors, a consistent theme emerged. The chief problem was that the manager expected the same strong work ethic that had led to his promotion to be present in his direct reports. Supervisors were expected to work 11–12 hours per day, and weekend staff meetings were routine. He unilaterally set aggressive goals for the department and made no effort to account for differences in managerial styles, personal preferences, or family responsibilities. In his mind, managers were to set direction and hold staff accountable for reaching the goals. Interestingly, he did not consider personal relationships when working toward results. The cycle of turnover continued unabated and eventually affected departmental performance to such an extent that it cost the manager his job. The manager had failed to recognize that his work expectations, though natural to him, were a stretch for many of his employees; consequently, he was unable to build effective relationships that would have contributed to sustained success for himself and the department as a whole. Perhaps more

(continued)

(continued from previous page)

important, he lacked the social and interpersonal skills that would have given him the insight to see what was happening.

Be mindful: Healthcare leadership is, at its core, a business of building and maintaining effective relationships with multiple and diverse stakeholder groups.

RELATIONSHIPS AS THE BASIS OF LEADERSHIP

From the dawn of the Industrial Revolution, the role of corporate managers in the United States evolved along task-oriented structures. The automotive industry developed leaders keenly adept at enhancing line productivity and focusing exclusively on objective metrics to be better, faster, and cheaper than competitors. Little or no attention was paid to staff satisfaction or retention. The prevailing attitude was captured in a quote sometimes attributed to Henry Ford: "Why is it every time I ask for a pair of hands, they come with a brain attached?" In response to the needs of the industrial base, business schools developed their curricula based primarily around objective competencies in the areas of finance, accounting, operational design, and marketing. These "hard skills" served as the basis for the master of business administration (MBA) degree, and they still make up the core curriculum of business education taught across the United States today.

In recent decades, however, more attention has been paid to developing the so-called "soft skills" in managers, as evidence has supported the link between positive relationships among leaders and staff and long-term organizational success. This shift in focus is a result of a variety of factors, including (1) the introduction into the workforce of new generations that demand a more participative leadership style and (2) the proliferation of technology and information sharing that allows companies to quickly adapt to changing trends in the business environment. Due to the latter influence, operational advances driven by the "hard skills" of management—such as improvements in productivity and processes that traditionally would have differentiated an organization among its peers—can quickly be discovered and replicated by others. Leaders have found, therefore, that the only sustainable competitive advantage is based on recruiting and retaining the very best people at all levels of the organization.

The ability to develop and sustain positive interpersonal relationships with staff has thus become a survival skill in an increasingly competitive war for talent, and nowhere is this competency more critical than in healthcare. Leaders in healthcare are in the business of managing highly trained and intelligent individuals, and these individuals are caregivers by nature who place a tremendous value on interpersonal relationships.

Although interpersonal skills are increasingly recognized as being critical to leadership success in healthcare, they are not an easy subject to teach, and their objective outcome metrics are difficult to quantify. As a result, many formal leadership development programs still do not have a significant focus on these skills. In fact, a study sanctioned by the American College of Healthcare Executives found that a significant percentage of senior executives rated recent graduates of healthcare leadership programs as being less prepared to effectively build and manage relationships than any prior generation of leaders. In addition, communication and interpersonal skills were among the lowest rated of all the key leadership competencies surveyed (Howard and Silverstein 2011). Results of the study, detailed in Exhibit 5.1, suggest that, even if the healthcare and business industries recognize the importance of maintaining effective relationships, organizations (and aspiring leaders) cannot rely on formal educational avenues alone to prepare managers for this fundamental task.

EXHIBIT 5.1: Senior Executives' Appraisal of Recent Healthcare Administration Graduate Competencies in Relation to Their Own Skills at the Same Stage

Competencies	Much Worse	Worse	About the Same	Better	Much Better
a. Managerial ethics and values	2 (1%)	45 (14%)	222 (72%)	36 (12%)	6 (2%)
b. Communication	8 (3%)	97 (31%)	136 (43%)	65 (21%)	9 (3%)
c. Problem solving	6 (2%)	87 (28%)	167 (54%)	44 (14%)	6 (2%)
d. Interpersonal skills	10 (3%)	82 (27%)	153 (50%)	56 (18%)	6 (2%)
e. Developing others	15 (5%)	106 (34%)	156 (50%)	35 (11%)	2 (1%)
f. Marketing/strategic planning	13 (4%)	101 (33%)	117 (38%)	60 (19%)	18 (6%)

Source: Reprinted with permission from Howard and Silverstein (2011).

The good news is that the competencies related to establishing and sustaining positive interpersonal relationships can be developed with the proper effort and attention. Some "natural leaders" might find these concepts more intuitive, but all leaders can enhance their skill sets and improve how they interact with those that they lead. In his groundbreaking book *Emotional Intelligence,* Goleman (1995) proposed that the science of building effective relationships as a leader begins with developing enhanced self-awareness (how well we know ourselves) and then evolves to an enhanced understanding of social awareness (how well we know and interact with others). Exhibit 5.2 illustrates the flow of emotional intelligence in three steps: gaining self-awareness, managing one's own emotions, and leading others.

Based on Goleman's work, many organizations now use selection criteria based not only on intelligence and problem-solving ability but also on the ability to relate to others effectively. In short,

EXHIBIT 5.2: Flow of Emotional Intelligence

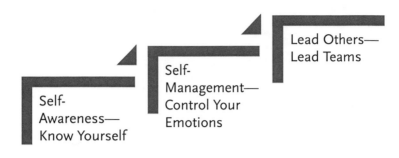

Self-
Awareness—
Know Yourself

Self-
Management—
Control Your
Emotions

Lead Others—
Lead Teams

they hold intelligence quotient, or IQ, and emotional intelligence quotient, or EQ, to be equally important in their hiring and promotional decisions. Though cognitive ability and IQ may be relatively fixed by genetics, emotional intelligence can be learned, practiced, and improved over time.

ENHANCING EMOTIONAL INTELLIGENCE

Goleman popularized five competencies of emotional intelligence that every business leader should work to develop: self-awareness, self-regulation, motivation, empathy, and social skills. In the protocol that follows, which is summarized in Exhibit 5.3, we have adapted and modified the key aspects of those competencies and applied them directly to the unique needs of leaders in healthcare.

EXHIBIT 5.3: Protocol for Enhancing Emotional Intelligence

Leaders should develop the following competencies to enhance emotional intelligence:

1. Improve self-awareness.
2. Practice self-regulation.
3. Hone your empathy and social skills.

Improve Self-Awareness

This competency refers to our ability to recognize and understand our own emotions, our personal strengths and weaknesses, and our tendencies to act in certain ways in given situations. Aristotle once said that "we are what we repeatedly do," and every leader has certain habits that have developed over time. Such habits result from operating within our own emotional "comfort zones" and having personal experiences that have shaped our management styles. Though these habits have a tendency to become embedded in our character, they can be recrafted with hard work. The first step is recognizing what habits have formed and which ones might act as barriers to effective relationships with those who work with and for us. Some practical strategies for enhancing self-awareness are outlined below:

- *Ask for feedback.* Leaders can get meaningful feedback on their leadership styles, strengths, and weaknesses through 360-degree evaluation systems. If a subordinate manager is leaving the organization, exit interviews can also provide helpful feedback; the individual might be more open with constructive criticism upon departure from the position. Leaders should be open to this feedback and use it as an opportunity to be self-reflective, rather than defensive.
- *Practice face-to-face interactions when possible.* Face-to-face interactions typically help minimize negative feelings and transform them into more positive relationships and outcomes. Such interactions also allow leaders to get real-time verbal and nonverbal feedback about their interpersonal skills. Body language and facial expressions can be positive or negative contributors to effective interpersonal connections.
- *Get out of your office.* Most individuals who work in a healthcare environment are caregivers by nature; thus

they place a high value on leaders who create strong interpersonal connections with staff and patients. Executives should practice rounding in a different unit of the hospital for 30 minutes each day, making a concerted effort to call staff by name, listening appreciatively to conversations, and envisioning themselves in the shoes and roles of the people with whom they speak. This practice, when done routinely, will serve to sharpen social awareness and enhance the leader's visibility in the organization.

Leadership Research and Theory Support

A significant number of research studies highlight the importance of interpersonal relationships in leadership success. One of the more pertinent is by Hogan and Kaiser (2005), who explore how strong leaders are able to promote highly effective team performance.

> Hogan, R., and R. B. Kaiser. 2005. "What We Know About Leadership." *Review of General Psychology* 9 (2): 169–80.

In another work in a similar vein, Hogan emphasizes that "The ability to do business depends on having a repertoire of social skills." Reviewing a US Department of Labor study that highlighted changing workplace competencies, he states, "The inclusion of interpersonal skills as a critical competency was a historic departure from traditional thinking, which focused solely on cognitive ability" (Hogan Assessments 2015, 1–2).

> Hogan Assessments. 2015. "Are You Employable? Interpersonal Skill in the Modern Job Market." Accessed October 6. www.hoganassessments.nl/uploads/file/Whitepapers/AreYouEmployable.pdf.

Practice Self-Regulation

The concept of self-regulation relates to our ability to manage emotions and impulses, maintain integrity in all interpersonal interactions, and take responsibility for our performance as leaders. Every middle school student recalls the experiments by Ivan Pavlov relating to stimulus and response: After a series of days in which he rang a bell before feeding his dogs, Pavlov discovered that the dogs would begin to salivate after the ringing of the bell even in absence of food being served; the salivating had become an instinctual response to a stimulus that the dogs had been trained to associate with food. As leaders, we must develop the ability to control our instinctual and emotional responses, and we must maintain a thoughtful and rational approach to interacting with others based on our internal values.

Controlling emotional responses can be difficult, but the following rules of thumb can help in forming more effective habits of self-regulation:

- *Be consistent.* Leaders should strive to be the same person every day, and to avoid vitriolic shifts in mood or temperament. In decision making, consistency is critical. Leaders should apply rules uniformly and should say and mean the same things to everyone in the organization, regardless of rank or power.

- *Deliver criticisms privately and constructively.* Although this concept seems basic, it often is violated, especially in staff meetings. Some leaders feel that if their criticism is not a formal disciplinary statement or if it is intended to provide motivation, then it can be delivered in front of peers. Some executives even feel that publicly delivered negative comments can serve as a rite of passage. In reality, messages delivered in this manner can be hurtful and demoralizing. Discussions around negative job performance should always be a thoughtful dialogue held in private.

- *Listen thoughtfully.* As a leader achieves a certain level of seniority and subordinates come to her with an issue, her initial response is often to solve the problem for them based on her own experiences in like situations. This approach not only stifles the subordinates' professional development, but it also can demoralize staff who may truly have just wanted to use the leader as a sounding board in the process of crafting their own solution. Leaders should make a point to spend more time in meetings *listening*—and allowing staff to be truly *heard*—rather than simply waiting for a chance to respond. Taking a few moments to listen helps to self-regulate emotional responses and provides time to craft a thoughtful dialogue internally.

Hone Your Empathy and Social Skills

Empathy—the ability to sense and respond to the feelings of others—is a key attribute in building effective interpersonal relationships. It is also, unfortunately, the quality that senior executives most often lack. Often, a leader tends to develop an attitude that, because of his position in the organization, those who work with and for him should simply alter their emotional responses to conform to his own. Such an attitude can be divisive and greatly reduce the chances that staff will be committed to the leader or the organization. Even if a leader is not a naturally empathetic person, a few simple tactics can help strengthen the ability to connect to others on a personal level:

- *Get to know your staff.* Caregivers and healthcare professionals are typically highly relationship driven.

A leader who knows about her subordinates' personal lives—their families, their personal interests—can develop a deeper understanding and concern, thus creating relationships that are stronger and that encourage loyalty.

- *Be personally vested in the success of others.* A leader's role should be to facilitate the success of the people working in the organization. Speak with the staff about the tools, training, information, and support they need to do their jobs well, and take action to remove any barriers to success.

- *Be tactful and diplomatic.* Always consider people's sensitivities—cultural, racial, and otherwise—in every interaction, and strive to honor their preferences.

- *Avoid favoritism.* Favoritism breeds dissention, resentment, and unhealthy competition. A healthcare delivery system is the ultimate team environment, and leaders need the full support of every employee. Leaders cannot be perceived as favoring one person over another.

- *Apologize gracefully, and forgive others.* Everyone occasionally makes errors or mistakes. When necessary, leaders should make amends for their mistakes with a direct and honest apology. Likewise, most employees will at some point make errors in judgment. Leaders do not have the luxury of holding grudges, and they should use mistakes as opportunities for coaching and professional growth.

SUMMARY

Leadership is a complex task that, by definition, relies on the engagement and actions of others. Though an individual leader can set a vision for the organization, that leader must leverage relationships with staff to execute the strategies necessary for achieving the vision. When relationships between leadership and staff are healthy, the vision ceases to be that of the leader solely; it becomes a shared understanding and collective excitement around what needs to be done to ensure the organization's success. In *The 7 Habits of Highly Effective People*, Covey (2013) likens the art of maintaining effective relationships to managing an "emotional bank account." Leaders must actively work to build equity with staff by making deposits in their account through thoughtful interactions and personal support. This positive equity can then be called on in difficult times when leaders must ask staff for sacrifices (e.g., working overtime during high-census periods, or going without an equipment upgrade when capital funds are scarce). By using the protocol outlined in this chapter, leaders can begin to build this precious equity with their staff and develop more effective personal habits to guide their interactions.

GUEST COMMENTARY: TIMOTHY P. ADAMS

I am often asked by young, aspiring healthcare leaders what it takes to be successful in this industry. Healthcare is admittedly a highly complex business requiring many skill sets, but I ultimately come back to one critical competency: relationship building. Your success will depend greatly on your ability to establish meaningful, sustainable relationships with your key constituents (patients, physicians, employees, the community, the board, fellow executive team members, and the list goes on). I have seen numerous executives—many of whom were highly intelligent, talented, well pedigreed, and capable of quickly analyzing financials and other operating metrics—ultimately fail because of their inability to effectively build

(continued)

(continued from previous page)

relationships. Conversely, I have seen many executives who were mediocre in their technical and financial skills but remarkable in their relationship skills go on to have successful careers.

Healthcare is fundamentally a service and relationship business. I consistently challenge our teams to be fully engaged in one critical mission: determining how to position our hospitals as the best places in our markets for employees to work, for patients to receive care, and for physicians to practice. If you can succeed in developing meaningful relationships with these three key groups—employees, patients, and physicians—you have a good chance of success as a healthcare executive.

I encourage you to seek out healthcare leaders who exhibit strong relationship-building skills. Closely watch how they engage with people and develop relationships, and then try to emulate their approaches. At the same time, take time to observe leaders who seem to have difficulty developing relationships. Sometimes you can learn as much from those who can't seem to build relationships as you can from those who do it well.

Timothy P. Adams
CEO, Central Region
Tenet Healthcare
Dallas, Texas

REFLECTIVE QUESTIONS

1. You work for a manager who is an introvert by nature and who does not feel comfortable interacting with staff. Though everyone respects his expertise and knowledge, they do not feel connected with him on a personal level. What initial steps might he take to begin building more effective relationships with his staff?

2. Take a moment to reflect upon your own leadership style. What emotions typically drive your decision making and interpersonal interactions? How do these emotional drivers change under times of stress?

3. What have you done in your career to determine your effectiveness with interpersonal relationships?

RESOURCES AND EXERCISES FOR LEADERSHIP DEVELOPMENT

1. If you have access to some of the style inventories (e.g., Myers-Briggs, Hogan Assessments), make time to take them and study their results. Ask others if they believe the results are descriptive of you.

2. If you have difficulty getting access to these style inventories, consider the following options:

   • David Keirsey and Marilyn Bates's book *Please Understand Me: Character and Temperament Types*, 5th ed. (San Diego, CA: Prometheus Nemesis Book Company, 1984) is widely available and provides a short Myers-Briggs Type Indicator survey.

   • The following websites have reputable interpersonal style questionnaires:

www.skillsyouneed.com/ls/index.php/343479/
www.psychometrictest.org.uk/interpersonal
    -skills-test/

REFERENCES

Covey, S. R. 2013. *The 7 Habits of Highly Effective People: Power-ful Lessons in Personal Change*, 25th anniversary ed. New York: Simon and Schuster.

Goleman, D. 1995. *Emotional Intelligence: Why It Can Matter More Than IQ*. New York: Bantam.

Howard, D. M., and D. Silverstein. 2011. "The Interpersonal Skills of Recent Entrants to the Field of Healthcare Management: Final Report." American College of Healthcare Executives. Published December. www.ache.org/pubs/research/Interpersonal -Skills-of-Recent-Entrants-v312-25-11.pdf.

PART II

Serving Others

CHAPTER 6

Engaging the Workforce

Employees who believe that management is concerned about them as a whole person—not just an employee—are more productive, more satisfied, more fulfilled. Satisfied employees mean satisfied customers, which leads to profitability.

—Anne M. Mulcahy, former CEO of Xerox

Guide to Reader

It is a simple but powerful precept: Leaders get things done through other people. Highly effective leaders are adept at getting employees engaged, enthused, and focused on the work at hand. We ask that readers be self-reflective as they read this chapter. To what extent do they view employees as simple instruments to get work done, as opposed to full-fledged partners in the mission of the organization? To what extent might leaders be abusing employees by not showing true respect? Success in leadership is evident when staff enthusiastically work toward the goals of the organization because of the personal equity their leader has built with them.

A Tale of Two Vice Presidents

Two department directors were promoted within their organization at approximately the same time as part of a formal restructuring and succession planning effort. Both individuals had risen through the management ranks quickly, with a long track record of successive promotions based on effective staff relationships and the ability to motivate others toward a common goal. When assuming their new roles, both were committed to not "losing touch" with the staff and frontline manager levels. They knew that, without the active engagement and support of these individuals, their tenure in the executive ranks might fall short of their lofty aspirations.

The first vice president went about networking and establishing relationships with his new executive peers and superiors within the C-suite. Because he had little formal interaction with these individuals during his time as a manager and department director, he felt he needed to spend a great deal of time getting to know them. Doing so would help him gain credibility and establish a new organizational identity as a hospital executive rather than a department head. His efforts proved to be fruitful, and he gained quick acceptance based on his insightful views and fresh perspective of hospital operations. However, as he celebrated his one-year anniversary in his first executive role, he began to hear rumblings that his managers and staff felt the move to vice president had "changed him" and that he was becoming "disconnected" from the staff. In response, he decided to participate in the hospital intramural softball league as a way to spend more time with staff away from the formal work setting. He had played on the radiology department team for three previous seasons, and his skill as

(continued)

(continued from previous page)

a former college baseball player helped propel the team to the hospital championship two years in a row. Because the current season was already nearly halfway over, he had to sign up as an alternate, and he was told he would be called if the team was short on players. In each of the six remaining games, several players were absent due to illness, injury, or family obligations, but the newly minted VP was never called to participate. After the season was over, he invited the department director to lunch and asked her why he had never been asked to play. Sheepishly, she admitted that most of the staff had said they just did not feel comfortable having an executive on the team, and that his presence would change the dynamics on the field. In this instant, the VP realized he had focused too much of his energies on relationship building with the executive team and not enough attention on maintaining an effective rapport with his staff.

The second vice president took a very different approach to her transition into the executive ranks. She was determined to not be viewed as another "suit" and to maintain strong relationships with the staff in her departments. She recalled that, when she began in her first manager role, she sponsored a weekly happy hour at a local sports bar so that she could build rapport with her staff in an informal setting. Looking to continue the practice, she issued an open invitation to all managers and staff that she would host a mixer every Friday evening to encourage team building. The events were well attended, the atmosphere was extremely informal, and conversation flowed freely after a few cocktails. The new VP accomplished her goal of getting to know her team on a personal level. Midway through the first year, however,

(continued)

(continued from previous page)

volumes in her departments began to lag. A competing healthcare organization had begun an aggressive marketing campaign around women's services, which was one of her key areas of responsibility, and the VP was forced to make quick and aggressive decisions to establish a new strategy to grow volume and cut expenses. She developed a plan she felt could put the departments back on a path for success, and she called a meeting of her department managers for discussion. But when she began the dialogue, she was met with an overarching attitude of apathy and resistance to change. She struggled to convince her management team of the need to alter the status quo. And because she had shared so many personal interactions with each of them, she felt uncomfortable initiating difficult conversations around their poor management performance in a time that required great change. In this moment, she realized that, though she had succeeded in keeping good personal relationships with her staff, she had allowed herself to become too "familiar" with them—they now struggled to view her as a leader.

Be mindful: The art of leadership, as in life, is fundamentally about balance. Leadership is a balance between task and relationship, and focusing too heavily on either side of the equation can limit the success of even the most talented executive. Leaders depend on effective relationships with staff to execute on the strategic objectives they have set out for the organization. However, these relationships must be developed and maintained within the appropriate professional boundaries, or else the executive risks losing credibility with the team. The protocols presented in this chapter are intended to assist leaders in striking the appropriate balance.

DEVELOPING A STAFF FOCUS

Management literature not only honors the importance of a dedicated and competent workforce but also recognizes that the success
of leaders rises and falls on the extent to which the staff supports
the mission and strategic objectives of the organization. In today's
rapidly changing healthcare landscape, organizations are serving an
aging population with an increased demand for services, while at
the same time dealing with shortages in the talent pool for many
key clinical disciplines. Under these circumstances, organizations
that are most effective at recruiting, retaining, and appropriately
motivating their workforce will have the greatest likelihood of
sustainable success. The ability to build good relationships with
managers and frontline staff is an essential part of the healthcare
leader's skill set. Certain cultural factors and commonly held stereotypes can serve as barriers to the development of effective staff
relationships, but every leader has the responsibility to recognize
and overcome these headwinds.

Because of differences in lifestyle, education, and socioeco-
nomic background, executives often feel they do not have much in
common with many of their employees. As a result, many senior
leaders are uncomfortable interacting with staff and often come
across as either awkward or overly "polished" in their presence. The
underlying social distinctions often become amplified in a work
setting and are reinforced by the formal organizational chain of
command. Hierarchies can emphasize power distinctions between
senior leaders and frontline staff, and these distinctions can seep
into the subconscious and affect the way we perceive one another.
No matter how approachable executives may be, some employees
will likely interact with them carrying preconceived notions that
the executives think too highly of themselves. Unfortunately, these
kinds of mental images can prevent many of us—executives and
staff alike—from getting to know one another, and they can bring
about discomfort and intimidation when we interact with people

with whom we do not typically socialize. Instead of learning how to rise above these feelings, many of us choose to avoid the interactions altogether.

Some executives are distant both in and out of the office setting, and they only spend time with their employees when they need something done. Consider, for instance, those CEOs who only go into the workplace when The Joint Commission arrives. In turn, some employees are equally distant and harbor ill will toward executives whom they perceive to be insincere. Once again, we see how perceptions can be more powerful than reality. More complicated interactions come into play when frontline staff members are promoted. Though this upward mobility is positive for the organization, interactions between the new leader and former colleagues can become strained if former peers perceive a change in behavior or interaction with the professional advancement.

Even in light of these challenges, many organizations have developed cultures that promote effective interactions between leaders and staff in both professional and social settings. Such successful interaction happens because both parties are open and willing to accommodate the other. Interaction should not appear unnatural; it should be considered part of a structured approach to developing effective staff relations on behalf of the executive. The protocol summarized in Exhibit 6.1 and described in the sections that follow can help leaders improve their working relationships with the rank and file.

EXHIBIT 6.1: Protocol for Developing a Staff Focus

The following framework can enhance the effectiveness of workforce interactions:

1. Turn the organizational chart upside down.
2. Give up the home field advantage.
3. Set the right tone.

Turn the Organizational Chart Upside Down

Leaders often tend to judge their worth by their title or by the scope of their organizational responsibility. The prevailing thought has been that the higher you move up in the organizational hierarchy, the more important and successful you have become. In a healthcare setting, however, those at the top of the organization are actually *least* positioned to have an impact on the *daily* operations of the organization. Though senior leaders can set large-scale standards and strategies, the caregivers are the ones who create the environment and outcomes. After all, patients will still receive care regardless of whether the CEO shows up to work. The key to long-term organizational success lies in engaging the hearts and minds of those on the front lines, so leaders should focus on empowering employees. They should seek to instill in employees a sense of personal pride in the organization and a sense of ownership for the organization's strategic objectives. In order to achieve this sense of ownership, leaders may have to avoid relying on their formal power and actively cede much of the authority for day-to-day operations to those closer to the patient experience. The following are some examples of how this shift in the balance of power can be manifested:

- *Appropriately delegate authority.* One of the most effective ways to show respect for employees' skill sets is to delegate the authority for important tasks, especially those tasks that directly affect employees' ability to perform their jobs. Healthcare organizations are notorious for requiring multiple levels of approval for even the most minor of expenditures. By contrast, Ritz Carlton luxury hotels have a policy that empowers any employee—from a front desk clerk with ten years of experience to a housekeeper brand new to the job—to address any need to enhance the customer experience, with the ability to spend up to

$2,000 without additional approvals! Not only does this policy facilitate rapid resolution of customer service issues; it also underscores to the employees that they are trusted to use their best judgment and that they "own" the goal of creating the ideal customer experience.

- *Be transparent.* For decades, people in leadership positions kept strategic information close to their vests. Many held a perceived notion that frontline employees would not understand or care about the complexities of the business world, or that the employees might share sensitive information that would compromise the organization's ability to execute on its goals. However, recent experience has shown the benefits of transparency for leaders as much as for caregivers. Caregivers who are open with patients and families when clinical errors are made have been found to have an improved chance of regaining trust and building ongoing relationships with the patients involved. Similarly, leaders who are open with staff about the organization's current performance (good or bad) and future direction can better educate the staff around the roles they can play in helping to achieve the established vision. Consider the current situation, in which the shifting reimbursement landscape has led many organizations down a path of significant cutbacks and reductions in force. Hospital leaders cannot control all of these dynamics, but they can provide regular updates to make the staff aware of how the organization is performing. The informed staff can then help devise creative solutions in times of reduced volume or reimbursement, perhaps offering ideas that will improve the organization's bottom line and save jobs. Too often, leaders take a paternalistic approach to problem solving and propose solutions without consulting the staff, even though frontline staff have the strongest grasp of the organization's daily operations. The perspective of the staff can only be obtained through an open environment that fosters communication and the sharing of information between executives and the front lines.

- *Be a facilitator, not a roadblock.* The role of a leader in an organization dedicated to employee engagement is one of collaboratively setting and communicating the organization's strategy and direction, creating a safe environment for staff to execute on this strategy (including allowing them to take calculated risks without fear of repercussions), providing the tools and support legitimately required for the work, and then removing any roadblocks (organizationally or environmentally) that could prevent the employees from doing their jobs effectively. Every executive should strive to be perceived by frontline staff not as a roadblock but as someone who works each day to ensure that the staff can provide the very best care to the patients served by the organization.

Give Up the Home Field Advantage

The concept of home field advantage comes from the sports world and states that teams tend to play better in their home stadium in front of a friendly audience and familiar surroundings. Similarly, business executives tend to fall into habits that reinforce the traditional power-based organizational hierarchy and cater more to their own preferences and comfort than to the convenience of the staff. Some of these habits have become so ubiquitous that leaders fail to consider how they might affect the staff; even actions leaders take to build positive relationships with the staff may, in fact, be having the opposite effect. In developing a culture of employee ownership, executives should remember that their position exists to improve the ability of the staff to perform their roles effectively—thus, leaders should always put the needs of the employees ahead of their own. Considerations include the following:

- *Abandon the open door policy.* For years, executives were taught that they needed to make themselves available to employees via an open door policy or a set time when employees can meet with the leader in the executive office. This policy, though noble in its intent, is symbolic of the traditional power-based management style in that it requires the employee to come to the manager rather than making the manager truly accessible to the employee. Some employees may feel comfortable going to the executive suite, but many more do not. In industry, many companies have chosen to locate the executive offices on the manufacturing floor as a forcing function, so that even the most senior leaders are required to interact with frontline staff daily (Graban 2012). Similarly, leaders in healthcare should spend time each day outside of their offices and actively seeking feedback from frontline employees.

- *Eat in the hospital cafeteria.* Time is the most precious commodity to every leader in healthcare, and the lunch break (when we are able to come up for air long enough to take lunch) can be a welcome respite in a fast-paced environment. Leaders often develop a habit of retreating to the office at lunchtime to catch up on e-mails or to try to make headway on the "to-do" list. The lunch hour, however, represents a wonderful opportunity to interact with the frontline staff in an appropriate social setting, and also to begin breaking down any "ivory tower" misconceptions people might have about elaborately catered meals in the executive suite. Take a few days each week to have lunch in the cafeteria, and sit with a group of employees rather than with other leaders. Lunch can provide an excellent platform for seeking feedback and providing updates on organizational performance.

- *Make off-shift visits.* Healthcare is a 24/7 business, and leaders are accountable not only for what happens on the day shift but also for what occurs after hours and on the weekends. The staff on the nighttime and weekend shifts often tend to feel disconnected from the happenings of the organization, and their lack of direct interaction and real information can contribute to misperceptions and rumors capable of poisoning the culture. Executives should regularly visit evening-shift employees by coming in early or staying late, and they should set a time to visit with staff on weekends. Coordinating the weekend visit with the week the executive is serving as the administrator on call can serve as a good reminder.

Leadership Research and Theory Support

Employee engagement has become a leadership mantra in recent years, and Men (2015) provides a broad review of the literature on the topic. She summarizes, "Employees perceive a better relationship with the organization when they perceive their managers to be authentic, ethical, balanced, fair, transparent, and consistent in what they say and do."

> Men, L. R. 2015. "Employee Engagement in Relation to Employee–Organization Relationships and Internal Reputation: Effects of Authentic Leadership and Transparent Communication." *Public Relations Journal.* Accessed October 6. www.prsa.org/Intelligence/PRJournal/Vol9/No2/.

Set the Right Tone

A leader's words and actions serve as cues to the employees about not only how the employees perceive the leader but also how they perceive the organization as a whole. Leaders may not always "feel" like a leader in every instance and circumstance; however, it is critical that they "act" the role of leader in all staff encounters to reinforce a culture of staff engagement. Leaders set the tone for the organization, and they must model the behavior and attitude they would like to see in the employees they are leading. Leaders are not allowed to have bad days, and if they do, they cannot make negativity evident to the employees. The following are some tips for setting a positive tone:

- *Be eternally optimistic.* Every organization will encounter difficult times, but exceptional leaders understand the importance of developing a strong strategy and exuding a positive outlook that the organization is on the right track. Similarly, leaders should always assume optimistic intent in terms of their interactions with others; they should not assume the worst about the motivations of their staff.

- *Do not complain.* Making negative comments about the performance of others—even if those comments are warranted—is typically counterproductive for those in leadership positions. First, it sends a message to the staff that complaining is an acceptable practice. Second, it might stoke animosity among employees who feel that executives are so well compensated that they should not be complaining about anything. Executives should remember that, in the eyes of the staff, the moment you become a victim, you cease to be a leader.

- *Adopt a can-do attitude.* Individuals who work to solve problems and find a way to collaborate with others have the ability to break through even the most burdensome bureaucracy.

SUMMARY

Healthcare is going through a period of great change, and change can be a frightening thing for employees who desire security and stability. It is often in periods of great change, however, that the most exciting innovations are developed. Our field is shifting from one centered on the provision of acute, episodic care to one that focuses the continuum of the patient experience in a customer-focused and high-quality manner. Transparency will become a hallmark of the future, with publicly reportable outcomes and quality data serving as a key driver of consumer decisions. Leaders within healthcare have the responsibility to engage the staff in their respective organizations not only to embrace these changes but also to see them as an opportunity—the chance to be part of an evolution that will greatly enhance the care provided to the patients they serve. In the years ahead, only those organizations that capture the creative energies of their employees and instill a sense of ownership within them will be able to make the transformative changes required without disrupting their current operations. The process will require a change in mind-set for leaders: Their vision of the executive role will shift from one of top-down decision making to that of a facilitator who delegates authority appropriately and empowers employees to help navigate the uncharted waters ahead.

REFLECTIVE QUESTIONS

1. Leadership is a balance between task and relationship. What are some risks of focusing too much on either driving results at all costs or being too familiar with your staff?

2. A strong link has been found between staff satisfaction and patient satisfaction. Why do you think this connection exists?

RESOURCES AND EXERCISES FOR LEADERSHIP DEVELOPMENT

1. Recent years have seen an increased focus on employee "engagement," as demonstrated by the fact that today's surveys are engagement surveys, not satisfaction surveys. Conduct some Internet research and determine (a) if there really is a difference between employee satisfaction and employee engagement, (b) what elements make up engagement, and (c) how employee engagement in your organization compares to the rates reported in articles found online.

2. Review the Human Resources Ethics Survey provided in Appendix A of this book. Complete the survey and use it as a basis for discussion with colleagues.

3. Read the *Harvard Business Review* article "Competing on Talent Analytics" (2010) by Davenport, Harris, and Shapiro, available here: https://hbr.org/2010/10/competing-on-talent-analytics. Do you agree with the primary tenets of the article?

4. The business strategy firm Root (www.rootinc.com) has based much of its employee engagement work on a quote:

   > Tell me, I'll forget. . . .
   > Show me, I'll remember. . . .
   > Involve me, I'll understand.

   The quote has been attributed to Benjamin Franklin but likely is originally from Xun Kuang, a Chinese Confucian philosopher who lived from 312 to 230 BC. How does this passage relate to your relationship with the workforce as a leader? And to what extent do employees have confidence that you are engaged with them in their work, versus directing them from the executive suite?

REFERENCE

Graban, M. 2012. *Lean Hospitals: Improving Quality, Patient Safety, and Employee Engagement.* New York: CRC Press.

CHAPTER 7

Executive Team Members

Just because you do not take an interest in politics doesn't mean politics won't take an interest in you.

—Pericles

Guide to Reader

Much of the focus on team building in management literature ignores the presence and impact of politics. However, office politics is omnipresent at the executive level and cannot be ignored. To be sure, politics is not all bad; it is simply a reality of day-to-day leadership work.

A Lesson in Office Politics

Tom was a long-standing CEO for a major market in a large, investor-owned hospital-operating company. He enjoyed a good rapport with his peers, built a strong reputation as a highly capable leader, and was held in high regard by the senior executive team within the organization. Because of his sustained track record of success, Tom was recently promoted into one of four regional CEO roles, giving him oversight responsibility for 15 hospitals in the southern United States. Although Tom is excited about the new position and the opportunity to have a broader impact within the organization, he quickly begins to have concerns about his working relationship with Connie, one of his peer regional CEOs.

Connie is a classic overachiever, having been promoted two years ago to run the northeastern region for the organization. Just 35, she became the youngest regional CEO in the history of the company. A Harvard MBA, she has earned a reputation for being bright and driven, but above all, she is known as the consummate politician. Connie has painstakingly ingratiated herself to all of her peers and to the senior leadership team, and she appears to have developed a collegial relationship with everyone in the executive suite—everyone, that is, except for Tom.

Tom and Connie have yet to connect on a personal or professional level, partially because of Tom's disdain for what he considers overly political maneuvering by Connie. Tom has observed that Connie interjects herself in areas that are not her responsibility in order to gain valuable information about broad corporate strategy outside her region. When such actions yield valuable information, Connie is selective

(continued)

(continued from previous page)

in how she shares the information she has gleaned. She provides in-depth information to colleagues she feels are supportive of her while offering minimal, if any, support to Tom. When her unsolicited information has a positive impact on the performance of her peer leaders, she is quick to share her contribution with their mutual supervisor, further positioning herself in a positive light as a "team player."

Tom has felt on several occasions that Connie purposely withheld vital information concerning best practices in her and other regions that could have proved beneficial in his own area of responsibility. Tom has approached his supervisor, the president of hospital operations, with his concerns but has received little support; Tom surmises that Connie's personal friendship has biased the president's decisions in Connie's favor. In addition, Connie has increasingly been receiving choice project assignments that are further raising her organizational profile, even though leadership of company-spanning projects is supposed to be equally distributed among the regional CEOs.

Tom continues to receive positive feedback from senior leadership, but the company has experienced two consecutive quarters of relatively poor financial performance. Tom worries that his position as the regional leader with the shortest tenure, in conjunction with Connie's passive–aggressive politics, might put his job at risk if any leadership cutbacks become necessary. Connie is well liked, extremely competent, and adept at positioning herself in a positive light, and she appears to have set her sights on Tom as a potential threat to her continued

(continued)

(continued from previous page)

upward climb. Tom is now in the unenviable position of trying to become more politically adept himself to combat what he perceives as a personal attack from a colleague.

Be mindful: Healthcare organizations are intensely political environments, and this atmosphere is often amplified in the executive offices. Conducting yourself in a professional and respectful manner at all times can help keep you out of the fray.

DEVELOPING A POLITICAL BALANCE

The hierarchical management structures in the organizations we lead have been created as systems of simultaneous competition and collaboration. These conflicting dimensions are embedded in the structures' design and clearly symbolized in organizational charts: The charts represent cooperation through their careful delineation and rational subdivision of tasks, but they also suggest potential conflict by displaying the career ladder on which people compete to ascend. Although competition for scarce resources is a reality in healthcare, the practice almost always has detrimental outcomes. The number of top positions in healthcare is finite, and the number of healthcare administrators vying for those roles is increasing almost daily. For leaders in our industry, the challenge is to be an effective advocate for oneself while minimizing competitiveness and maintaining camaraderie and personal relationships with competitive peers. This balance is an art form that requires portions of confidence, humility, aggressiveness, and appropriate restraint. Roberto (2013) writes that leaders must "cultivate constructive conflict in order to enhance the level of critical and divergent thinking, while simultaneously building consensus in order to facilitate the timely and efficient implementation of the choices

EXHIBIT 7.1: The Delicate Act of Balancing in the C-Suite

Conviction and assuredness	Meekness and modesty
Aggressiveness and forcefulness	Moderation and mild-manneredness
Directives	Collaboration and consensus

they make." Simply put, this is not easy. Leaders may benefit from visualizing the balancing act as it is portrayed in Exhibit 7.1.

In the vignette from the beginning of the chapter, Connie might be described as an overachiever, and her behavior might be characterized as overly political. Though she may not be doing anything unethical, she has made a habit of focusing primarily on her own position in the organization even if it means withholding information that might help a colleague. Tom, on the other hand, could be described as apolitical. Until he felt an immediate threat, he seemed content to allow Connie to maneuver and did little to convince his peers and superiors of the value he could add to the organization. In short, Connie and Tom represent opposite ends of the leadership balance.

Effective and upwardly mobile leaders tend to develop an "appropriate boldness." Essentially, this concept involves finding a point that avoids unethical behavior but involves striving to make sure others in the organization see your handprint. Building an effective professional network, avoiding marginalization, and cultivating a positive organizational identity are all priorities worth pursuing; however, an equilibrium must be maintained. Over time, being either overpolitical or underpolitical can derail a promising career. The protocol presented in this chapter is intended to assist healthcare leaders in striking the right balance.

BARRIERS TO EFFECTIVE OFFICE POLITICS

Before we discuss how to appropriately network within the executive suite, we should examine two common products of unhealthy competition: jealousy and tunnel vision. Both need to be actively mitigated to establish an appropriate political climate. If left unchecked, they can create team friction and have a destructive impact on executive team dynamics and the organization's well-being.

Jealousy

Jealousy is the product of unhealthy rivalry between individuals, and it frequently appears when unequal standards for recognition and rewards are perceived. The following are some areas in which jealousy can take root:

- *Organizational reporting structure.* Executives oftentimes define worth or influence based on the person to whom a position reports in the company hierarchy. A senior executive reporting to the CEO, for instance, might be viewed by peers as having more direct influence and a higher status than a leader who has a reporting line to the COO.

- *Title inflation.* In the quest to create career tracks for the leadership ranks, organizations have introduced a host of new titles, such as *senior director, associate vice president, senior vice president,* and *executive vice president.* Though the scope and responsibility associated with these titles can vary widely from one organization to another, the trend has fostered expectations of title elevation among many healthcare leaders. Such expectations can lead to jealousy or friction within the executive team if titles are not assigned judiciously.

- *Scope of responsibility.* Many leaders in healthcare strive to gain the broadest span of control possible in their organizations, as defined by the number of departments, facilities, or full-time equivalent (FTE) employees for which they have oversight responsibility. Top executives who distribute responsibilities among their executive team members need to be mindful of possible implications for team dynamics. Inequitable distribution can send an unspoken message of favoritism and create unwarranted tension.

- *Organizational resources.* Allocation of organizational resources—such as funding for FTEs or capital equipment—is a particularly sensitive issue, because every healthcare organization has needs that outstrip the available budget. If one executive is perceived as receiving more than his "fair share," jealousy can develop.

Certain tactics can help reduce the threat of jealousy in the executive suite. Feelings of jealousy often arise from misperception or poor understanding of organizational priorities and the responsibilities of other executives in the company. Thus, the best way to minimize jealousy is to create an environment in which all the executives fully understand and appreciate one another's roles. Consider, for instance, having an open executive committee meeting in which major funding decisions and capital allocations are discussed, asking all members of the executive team (even nonclinical leaders) to take administrative call, and rotating backup responsibility among team members when one executive is out on vacation. Such actions can foster a greater appreciation for the challenges each member of the team faces on a daily basis.

Tunnel Vision

Tunnel vision is the tendency to view the organization through a single lens, essentially discounting the importance or validity of the needs of other parts of the organization. Healthcare might be more prone to tunnel vision than any other industry. General businesses have created leadership development programs in which emerging leaders have rotational experiences through several functional areas in order to create a generalizable skill set. Such practices are rare in healthcare. Leaders in healthcare are often the product of progressive promotion through a single specialist track, such as nursing, ancillary services, or facility administration. Even those executives who have served in a variety of leadership roles often do not gain exposure to functional areas such as human resources, information technology, or marketing until they are already in a very senior role, such as CEO or COO; essentially, they are in the position of having to learn on the job. It is critical, therefore, that when an organization is facing major decisions—such as financial cutbacks, strategic planning, or budgeting—the top leaders not allow the executives to resort to protecting their "turf." Instead, the executives should be encouraged to take broader perspectives and make decisions that benefit the entire organization, even if the positive effects of those decisions might be felt more prominently in areas outside their scope of responsibility.

EFFECTIVE EXECUTIVE TEAM INTERACTIONS

Although these barriers might prompt some executive team members to develop an overly political or siloed approach, the most effective leaders develop behaviors that engender collaborative relationships while still advancing their own political agendas. The following protocol, which is summarized in Exhibit 7.2, is designed to improve interaction among leaders and, in turn, increase the overall effectiveness of the organization.

EXHIBIT 7.2: Protocol for Effective Office Politics

The following framework can enhance the effectiveness of executive team interactions:

1. Communicate persuasively.
2. Don't be afraid to celebrate your successes.
3. Encourage healthy conflict.
4. Understand the political climate.
5. Establish accountability.
6. Play politics the right way.
7. Set up organizational "rules of engagement."

Communicate Persuasively

As evidenced in the vignette at the beginning of the chapter, trying to attain power and influence by withholding information and trading the information for personal gain can seriously jeopardize teamwork. Competent executives foster an environment of open communication and sharing of information. Leaders should develop assertive communication styles backed by solid facts and examples. The most politically savvy leaders manage their messages to meet the key needs of various audiences; doing so enables them to become trusted sources of information to all constituencies. Nonetheless, these leaders are also careful not to align themselves with any one group too strongly. Political pressures can pit one group against another, so leaders should strive to be trusted advisers to all and steer clear of potentially fleeting alliances or office coalitions.

Don't Be Afraid to Celebrate Your Successes

If your good work goes unnoticed, you run the risk of having others take credit for your results and losing in the game of office politics when you really deserve to win. Take regular opportunities to let your supervisor know about key successes and the value you have brought to the organization. At the same time, be careful to maintain a semblance of humility: Do not exaggerate your contributions or come across as a braggart, and always recognize the work of others when the success was a team effort.

Encourage Healthy Conflict

Peter Senge (2006) proposed in his groundbreaking work on organizational dynamics, *The Fifth Discipline*, that the most effective leadership teams possess a healthy amount of conflict. He maintains that this conflict—which he describes as "creative tension"—actually encourages effective dialogue and results in improved strategic decision making. A certain amount of controversy and confrontation should be encouraged as long as participants maintain a professional manner and do not sink to personal attacks. Healthy conflict helps ensure that all concerns are surfaced and all team members have the opportunity to work through any doubts or reservations they may have.

When engaging in conflict with peers, be careful not to allow your words or actions to cross into areas that might be perceived as unethical. In the heat of the moment, the lines between effective politicking and office sabotage can blur quickly, so leaders should have a mental checklist that they go through when they engage with colleagues. According to guidelines by the Center for Business Ethics at Bentley College (2014), leaders assessing the ethics of a specific decision, action, or political tactic should consider the following questions:

- Is it right?
- Is it fair?
- Who gets hurt?

- Would you be comfortable if the details of your decision or actions were made public in the media or through e-mail?
- What would you tell your child, sibling, or young relative to do?
- How does it smell?

Understand the Political Climate

To further your understanding of the political climate, observe how tasks get accomplished in your organization and determine how and why some leaders are more successful than others in advancing their agendas. Ask key questions about the organization: What are the core values and how are they enacted? What is the organization's tolerance for risks? Which leadership behaviors are rewarded, and which have been discouraged? Once you have a grasp of the overall leadership culture, try to understand the dynamics of your executive team. If you sense any office turmoil directed at you, strive to resolve the issues quickly; if needed, discuss them in private with your boss rather than taking retaliatory actions. By understanding the political environment and knowing what behavior is tolerated and rewarded in your organization, you can avoid political blunders that could taint your organizational identity.

Establish Accountability

The assignment of responsibility helps ensure that a task gets done. However, it also creates the opening for two potential conflicts that can surface in teamwork: The first arises when too many leaders want responsibility for a high-profile project, and the second arises when no leaders want accountability for a project because it is considered menial or has a low probability of success. The CEO or COO should fairly and rationally distribute accountability for all projects, and executives should feel comfortable advocating for leadership of the specific projects they desire. In their advocacy efforts, however, leaders should focus on how their individual skill sets align with what will be required to successfully execute the project, rather than on attacking the competency of other leaders who may be competing for the same project.

Play Politics the Right Way

Leaders often make the bold statement, "I simply do not play politics"—but perhaps the real crux of the matter is the definition of "playing politics." Without spending a lot of time and space chasing that definition, suffice it to say that everyone in a group setting interacts with one another, and the interactions often deal with matters of power and influence, titles, ambition, and potential conflict. We could argue that any participation in these interactions amounts to playing politics. But we would also point out that some approaches to these interactions are more appropriate than others. Playing politics the right way typically involves the following elements:

- *Truth telling.* Leaders are wise to always tell the truth. Often, leaders work in environments where few outright lies are told but where facts are misconstrued to give the slight appearance of deceit. Effective leaders ferret out these situations before they aggregate and grow into serious problems.
- *Emphasizing the organizational mission.* A common goal or a common threat often serves to unify a group. Consistently listing the organizational mission as a common cause can help keep conflicts down and the focus on the future.

- *Building relationships based upon respect.* Consultants in team building indicate that respect among members is an absolute requirement for team effectiveness.
- *Avoiding hyperbole.* Exaggeration is perhaps the single biggest cause of small organizational friction and can lead to serious problems in closely working teams.
- *Finding common ground.* Building personal connections with others can improve interactions in much the same way a common organizational mission can. Gaining personal insight into fellow team members helps you understand their goals, interests, and concerns. Leaders should make time throughout the year to socialize out of the workplace and discuss nonwork matters.
- *Being willing to admit being wrong.* Some leaders feel that admitting one's mistakes is a sign of weakness. In fact, the opposite is true, and all leaders should adopt this principle early in their careers and continue to sustain it throughout.

Set Up Organizational "Rules of Engagement"

Teams that work well together have rules of engagement that seek to minimize the negatives of playing politics. Whereas most teams have unwritten rules and expectations, the more sophisticated teams actually develop the rules as a group, discuss them, and commit them to writing. Even if the written rules seem simplistic, a team can benefit from having guides on how the group makes decisions, how members conduct business in and out of meetings, how the team formalizes agreements, and how it manages conflict. Many teams begin the rule-making process by addressing less complex matters, such as sending materials for review in advance of meetings, preparing agendas, and using minutes for tracking accountability. As teams get deeper into the processes, the rules

EXHIBIT 7.3: Sample Rules of Engagement—Southern Ohio Medical Center

- We work hard on things that matter.
- We select the right leaders for the right jobs.
- We concentrate on asking the right questions.
- We avoid secrecy.
- We embrace discomfort.
- We talk to each other, not about each other.
- We grow thick skins.
- We hold each other accountable.
- We make our expectations clear.
- We set high expectations for ourselves and others.
- We listen more than we talk.
- We deal with conflict directly and resolve it promptly.
- We examine our options, deliberately choose the best one, and then act without undue delay.
- We face reality.
- We take full responsibility for our own feelings and behaviors.
- We deliver on our commitments.
- We recognize that emotional arousal is a danger sign.
- We build lasting relationships by engaging in real work as a team.
- We cut each other some slack—but not too much.
- We have fun.

Source: Southern Ohio Medical Center (2003).

become more sophisticated. Exhibit 7.3 provides an example of one organization's rules of engagement.

SOME GENERAL SUGGESTIONS

We conclude this chapter with the following general suggestions for maintaining positive interactions among the executive team:

- Be cautious with the use of e-mail: It can be a time saver, but it can also be detrimental to personal interaction. Opportunities to converse in a give-and-take manner, to observe body language, and to clarify misunderstandings are lost in e-mail exchanges.

- Speak objectively. Much personal conflict results from people either speaking in platitudes or using dramatic subjectivity in their language. Avoid emotional statements and exclamations—for instance, "Oh, come on," or "No one would even dream of this," or "Literally every single doctor in the group favors this"—that are likely to escalate the conflictual nature of a debate.

- Build alliances, but do so carefully. People group together—this is a fact—but some relationships run deeper than others. Teams that work together most effectively are ones that can minimize the dissonance from cliques that form within them.

- Be assertive.

- Become comfortable saying, "I don't know." So many leaders fall prey to giving rushed, inaccurate answers to questions raised in meetings or making up "facts on the fly" when talking to groups. Often, the better option is to simply say, "I don't know, but I'll check."

- Learn the art of compromise and win–win.

SUMMARY

Healthcare organizations are highly political entities by nature. Though some leaders prefer not to participate in or even think about office politics, learning how to effectively navigate these potentially dangerous waters can be critical to long-term success. A leader's political savvy can significantly help or hinder the ability to get things done. Office alliances can be fleeting, but the best leaders are able to build and maintain effective relationships with peers even in a highly competitive environment. In negotiating office politics, leaders should make the professional decision to be responsible and honest. Those who make passive–aggressive comments or actively seek to undermine the decisions of others are typically insecure in their ability to compete on their own merit. Through rational and steady leadership, you can advance your career ethically and become a trusted resource for your boss and peers alike.

GUEST COMMENTARY: J. MARK MCLOONE

A truly great leader possesses the emotional maturity to realize that the creation of an organization that will grow and thrive, even after that leader is gone, is the ultimate expression of success. Guiding a team to support a culture that leads to the development of such an organization requires both a tolerance for "dynamic tension"— which produces better decisions—and the skill to lead discussions toward positive results.

This dynamic tension requires diversity of opinion, experience, and skill amongst the team members. Diversity must be considered from the beginning of the recruitment process of the team members. The leader must foster a culture that supports the freedom to express the differences of opinion that such diversity infuses. Perhaps most important, the leader must ensure an atmosphere of mutual respect so that all members of the team know that their input is valued, regardless of how popular their opinions may be.

Individual representatives of the team will bring differing views to a particular issue. The optimal decision or outcome is achieved when the team arrives at a collective

(continued)

(continued from previous page)

agreement, which can be an exhausting and time-consuming process. Bringing such a diversity of viewpoints to a common, best decision or outcome often requires reviewing enough data or varied experiences to build a shared understanding. Ultimately, however, the mutual understanding of the team members and the decisions resulting from the process lead to a level of performance excellence that rewards all those who participate.

The authors present an interesting case in the vignette that begins this chapter, and we might ask ourselves how the individuals described rank the importance of creating an organization with sustainable excellence compared with the importance of their own personal achievement. How would you mentor them to facilitate the establishment of such an organization of sustainable excellence?

J. Mark McLoone
Chief Executive Officer
St. Christopher's Hospital for Children
Philadelphia, Pennsylvania

REFLECTIVE QUESTIONS

1. If you were Tom in this chapter's vignette, how would you approach your relationship with Connie? Would you work around her, confront her, or seek to develop an alliance?

2. Think of a time in which you were the victim of office politics. How could you have used the protocol in this chapter to manage a more positive outcome?

RESOURCES AND EXERCISES FOR LEADERSHIP DEVELOPMENT

1. Many "political" problems occur because all, or practically all, of the interactions among the team members occur in the work setting. As a result, team members often know one another only professionally. If you have the authority or influence to do so, schedule some type of team activity outside the normal scope of work (and out of the physical workplace) to allow team members to get to know one another on a personal basis.

    A variety of Internet resources can help you plan such an activity:

    *   One of the better sites for team exercises is from Mind Tools: www.mindtools.com/pages/article/newTMM _52.htm.

    *   Some getaway activities can be built around setting team rules and determining how the team is to interact. See www.workshopexercises.com/team_building _continued.htm for information.

    *   An excellent team questionnaire can be found at www .mindtools.com/pages/article/newTMM_84.htm.

2. The Rules of Engagement from the Southern Ohio Medical Center, shown in Exhibit 7.3 and available at www.somc .org/employee/assets/press/RulesOfEngagement.pdf, provide an excellent guide for team behavior. Set aside time with your team to review the full copy of the document and use it as a springboard for discussion. Consider developing your own rules for engagement for your team.

REFERENCES

Bentley College Center for Business Ethics. 2014. "Guidelines for Ethical Decision Making." Accessed April 1. www.bentley.edu /cbe.

Roberto, M. A. 2013. *Why Great Leaders Don't Take Yes for an Answer: Managing for Conflict and Consensus*, 2nd ed. Upper Saddle River, NJ: FT Press.

Senge, P. M. 2006. *The Fifth Discipline: The Art and Practice of the Learning Organization*. New York: Doubleday.

Southern Ohio Medical Center. 2003. "Rules of Engagement: Some Expectations for SOMC Leaders." Published June. www .somc.org/employee/assets/press/RulesOfEngagement.pdf.

CHAPTER 8

The Governing Board

The chief executive officer who avoids seeking the advice of directors regarding management practices is acting unwisely, if not imprudently. Presidents and other top-echelon managers may use the board as a voice of conscience, a control mechanism, a sounding board, or an endorsing agent, but they should use it.

—James L. Hayes

Guide to Reader

Interactions with board members carry many rules, traditions, and customs. The ability to understand the tact and discretion that overlap these exchanges is a function of great insight and artful finesse. Incorporating skills that are often not developed until much later in one's career, the protocol presented in this chapter is among the most challenging to learn and most difficult to master.

The Buck Stops Here

On a bright summer day in a former gold-mining boom
town, an 18-year-old star athlete is participating in the first
organized football practice of his senior season. Coming
off a year in which he set the state record for passing
yards by a quarterback (a record that had stood for more
than 20 years), he and his coaches have their sights set
on bringing home the first state football title in the small
town's history. Midway through what had been a relatively
uneventful practice, the young quarterback drops back to
pass and, just as he releases the ball, is hit in the right leg
by an overly aggressive freshman defensive end. An audible
crack is heard, followed by the sight of glistening white
bone protruding from the shin. Knowing that their star has
been seriously injured, the coaching staff personally rush
him to the local community hospital, which is only three
blocks away.

Once they arrive at the Emergency Department, an X-ray
quickly confirms that the quarterback has suffered a
fractured fibula, and the nursing staff calls for the physician
to assess the situation. The emergency room physician
evaluates the patient nearly an hour later, and rather than
calling the orthopedic physician on call (which would
have been standard protocol), he decides that his years of
experience have given him the necessary background to set
and cast a small bone fracture such as this one. Though
the nurses find this decision strange, they do not question
it. The physician proceeds to set and cast the bone while
in the emergency department, and he discharges the
quarterback home with instructions to return in six weeks
to get the cast removed.

(continued)

(continued from previous page)

On three separate occasions over the next week, the patient calls the hospital complaining about pain in his leg and the cast "smelling funny." A prescription for oral pain medication does not improve his symptoms, so the physician asks him to come back to the emergency department for an evaluation. When the cast is removed, the staff is shocked to see that the leg has developed a gangrenous infection that requires immediate amputation below the knee.

The ensuing lawsuit reveals that the emergency room physician was a moonlighting doctor who had only been at the hospital for a couple months and that his credentials had been hastily approved by the board of trustees on the recommendation of the CEO, in an effort to fill gaps in coverage. The doctor had an extensive malpractice history that only came to light after his credentials had already been approved, and his privileges as an emergency room physician did not include the approval to apply casts for broken bones (a fact of which the emergency room staff were well aware). Given this information, the quarterback's family not only sued the hospital but also sought personal damages from each member of the board of trustees for lack of oversight.

Be mindful: Governing board members in healthcare organizations have assumed great responsibility, and they willingly devote their personal time to help make the facilities they serve a better and safer environment for patient care. Healthcare leaders should respect this sacrifice and make every effort to provide the tools, education, and communication necessary to support trustees in their efforts.

THE EVOLVING ROLE OF BOARD OVERSIGHT

In the early days of healthcare administration in the United States, appointees to hospital boards of directors carried little responsibility. Influential community members and civic leaders chose to serve either out of a sincere desire to improve their community or to advance their social standing. Hospitals were seen simply as places where physicians chose to practice their craft, and the management of a facility bore little, if any, responsibility for the quality of care delivered by those physicians. In the summer of 1965, however, this view changed significantly. In the landmark case of *Darling v. Charleston Community Memorial Hospital*, a court found in favor of a young quarterback who had lost his leg to a negligent doctor who was allowed by a hospital board of directors to practice without appropriate oversight or vetting. The case, which inspired the vignette that begins this chapter, started the evolution of the modern board's fiduciary responsibility in healthcare organizations. This fiduciary responsibility has since expanded to include the financial health of the organization as well as the standards and quality of care provided.

Today, case law clearly states that healthcare directors are subject to personal financial and civil penalties for lapses in oversight, and additional factors within the industry are changing the way boards of directors function. Recent healthcare reform laws have ushered in a new era of transparency for the industry. Quality metrics, patient satisfaction scores, and outcomes data are now public information, and they apply new pressure on hospital management teams and directors to understand not only the data but also the underlying processes contributing to the hospital's current performance and the actions being taken to improve them. Davidson and Murdock (2013) write, "In light of the federal government's increased emphasis on regulatory compliance and False Claims Act enforcement, this responsibility should not be taken lightly." Taken together, advances in quality measurement and public reporting require boards of healthcare institutions to focus not only on financial performance but also on quality; an insufficient focus on the latter can lead to the loss of direct financial incentives, potential reputational harm, and a negative impact on market share and consumer choice.

Courts of law, governmental regulatory agencies, and accrediting bodies (such as The Joint Commission) now uniformly look to the governing board as the ultimate authority on the operations of a healthcare organization. Though this authority is broad and takes many forms, the basic responsibilities of the governing board can be summarized in four core areas:

1. *Preserving the institution's assets.* A hospital is a key community resource, and the board of directors bears the ultimate responsibility for managing the finances of the organization in a manner that will ensure its ongoing survival. This responsibility involves overseeing the overall financial condition, ensuring the appropriateness and legality of contractual agreements, obtaining adequate business and liability insurance coverage, preventing and guiding through regulatory or legal entanglements, and setting internal capital and external investment strategies. Most boards perform these functions through committees made up of appropriate trustee content experts. For example, financial activity is reviewed through the board finance committee, which comprises community trustees with specific expertise in finance, business, and accounting.

2. *Ensuring quality of care.* This responsibility now goes well beyond the traditional mechanisms of reviewing and approving the credentials of physicians prior to granting them practice privileges in the institution. In an era of enhanced transparency, trustees are expected to be well versed on the organization's quality plan, to review and approve all quality-related policies and procedures, to understand the organization's performance

improvement initiatives, and to ensure compliance with care-related regulatory statutes, such as medical necessity requirements, the False Claims Act, and the Emergency Medical Treatment and Active Labor Act (EMTALA). This responsibility presents a daunting proposition to even the most informed and dedicated lay trustee. The National Quality Forum (2004) conducted a survey of healthcare trustees across the United States and concluded that "board members often express confusion and uncertainty about what exactly they need to do to fulfill their responsibilities to oversee healthcare quality." This dynamic should be recognized and actively addressed by hospital leadership through ongoing trustee education.

3. *Appointing the organization's CEO.* Because the trustees are often community volunteers with their own jobs and interests, they delegate their oversight authority in day-to-day practice to the organization's CEO and management team. The selection of the CEO is perhaps the most important decision a board makes. Choosing the right CEO—and understanding the strengths and weaknesses of the senior leadership team the CEO puts together—can be the difference between organizational success and failure. In addition, with all the changes sweeping the healthcare field and CEO turnover near an all-time high (American College of Healthcare Executives 2015), the board must have formal succession plans in place for the CEO and other management positions.

4. *Overall fiduciary responsibility.* This all-encompassing duty essentially means that because the board legally has the ultimate authority on all functions of the organization, it also is ultimately liable for all the organization's decisions.

All healthcare leaders should understand this summary of board responsibilities, because it explicates the tremendous demands placed on board members and signals the areas in which power struggles between the chief executive officer and board members can develop. Immediate causes of power struggles may include institutional bureaucracy, personality conflict, varying management views, and differences over strategic direction. However, the roots of such struggles can often be traced to poor communication and a lack of effective working relationships. The guidelines presented in this chapter focus on building a well-functioning board and maintaining strong working relationships between the leadership team and trustees. The recommendations are aimed primarily at CEOs, who have a high level of interaction with trustees, but they also provide useful guideposts for other leaders and those who aspire to become CEOs.

EFFECTIVE BOARD INTERACTIONS

The role of the board in healthcare has morphed from one of pure oversight into one with an expanded management function, particularly in the areas of finance, compliance, and quality. For trustees to execute this function effectively, the board must have a symbiotic relationship with the hospital executive team, and the relationship must move the organization toward its ultimate goal of providing safe, high-quality, and efficient care. The following protocol, which is summarized in Exhibit 8.1, aims to improve interaction among executives and trustees and, in turn, increase the overall effectiveness of the organization.

EXHIBIT 8.1: Protocol for Effective Board Relations

The following framework can enhance the effectiveness of executive team and trustee interactions:

1. Build a great board.
2. Arm the board with information.
3. Establish effective board relationships.
4. Manage the board wisely.
5. Regularly review board functionality.

Build a Great Board

Just as a chef's signature dish is only as good as the ingredients used, a CEO cannot expect to have a high-functioning board unless great care has been taken to select trustees with the appropriate expertise, interests, leadership philosophy, and attitude. Leaders should commit to the following guidelines when assembling or replacing members of the board:

- *Participate in the screening and selection of board members.* A seat on the board of a healthcare organization is no longer an honorary position. It should not be offered as a reward to those who donate significant amounts of money to the organization but rather to those whose skills and ideas can advance the organization's strategic mission. Serving as a trustee in today's healthcare environment is both challenging and time consuming, and candidates right for the job must be prepared to spend a great deal of effort learning and orienting themselves to the industry. A CEO should be as deeply involved as possible in suggesting and screening prospective board members. After all, the CEO's own success may ultimately be decided by how well new board members can assist in the execution of the organization's strategy.
- *Manage conflicts of interest.* The key to protecting against conflicts of interest among board members is to establish a written policy that deals with such issues. The policy should identify potential sources of conflict of interest and enumerate the subsequent actions that will be taken if such conflicts are discovered. You cannot guarantee that board members will not use their positions for personal gain; however, a well-written policy can help protect the organization in case those situations occur.

- *Select members who can truly help the organization.* The responsibilities of the board are broad and far-reaching, so the makeup and expertise of the trustees should be reflective of these demands. An overly homogenous board might lack the diversity of viewpoints needed to address all the various issues that may arise; thus, trustees should be selected from a variety of social, professional, and racial backgrounds. CEOs should also be aware of their own professional weaknesses and select trustees who can help provide guidance in those specific content areas.

- *Do not hire relatives of board members.* Nepotism, or any variation of it, is a harmful business practice that can lead to numerous problems, even beyond the obvious perceptions of favoritism. The leadership team will be in a difficult situation if it needs to terminate the relative of a board member after the relative has proved to be a poor fit for the position. Moreover, relatives of board members often may parlay their relationships in inappropriate ways. One tip is especially important in this matter: Ideally, the board, rather than the CEO, should initiate and approve the policy dealing with nepotism.

Arm the Board with Information

Many trustees who serve on boards come from industries outside of healthcare, and they may have little or no baseline knowledge of the standards and oversight for which they are now responsible. Hospital leaders therefore must educate their board members and develop a transparency that keeps the members informed of the key issues facing the organization. The following actions can help to ensure the success of healthcare trustees:

- *Provide ongoing education.* According to a National Quality Forum (2004) report, most healthcare trustees feel ill-prepared to execute their fiduciary responsibilities, particularly in the area of quality. Providing regular opportunities for meaningful education is thus an important step in developing and maintaining positive relationships and increasing the overall effectiveness of the board. Too often, leaders mistakenly assume that meaningful board education must involve formal retreats with high-priced outside speakers. To the contrary, many boards have found greater success by dedicating 30 minutes at the beginning of each board meeting for internal experts (e.g., functional leaders, physicians, or executive team members) to present a topic of interest or to lead an in-depth discussion on a particular strategic matter. The more educated board members are about the industry, the organization, and the key issues the leadership team is facing, the more likely they are to be a positive and supportive force to the CEO.

- *Share information completely and immediately.* Formally, informally, collectively, and individually, effective communication between the CEO and trustees is essential. The board can only perform its duties if its members are well informed of what is going on. Mechanisms should be in place to guarantee the adequate flow of information among board members and between board members and the CEO. Key information should be communicated in advance of formal meetings, and any potentially damaging news should be shared immediately. Surprises are not appreciated by board members and can often be career limiting for executives.

- *Declare and communicate failures quickly.* Trustees do not expect leaders in the organization to be infallible. Innovation is essential for success in a rapidly changing healthcare environment, and an emphasis on innovation will likely lead to some strategic bets not playing out as anticipated. In these instances, the board (or appropriate committee) should be informed of failures and of the lessons the leadership team has learned to ensure better performance going forward.

Establish Effective Board Relationships

As with any working or personal relationship, the success of interactions between executives and trustees is directly proportionate to the energy that both sides devote to building effective relationships with each other. The following actions can help create strong board–executive partnerships:

- *Create trust.* Trusted alliances are critical, and CEOs should devote time on a regular basis to developing personal connections with each member of the board. Successful CEOs have shared that they benefit from meeting with trustees one-on-one rather than relying on group sessions. The unwavering relationships that result can transform the board into a network of trusted advisers with whom the CEO can confide during the most difficult of situations.

- *Encourage direct relationships with management staff.* Though formal communications to the board should always be coordinated through the office of the CEO, the CEO should not consider herself a filter between the staff and the board. Open access between the board and the leadership team can help trustees assess the health of the organization from different perspectives. This open-access approach also demonstrates the confidence the CEO has in her own abilities and in her relationships with the board and the executive team.

- *Respect board members' time and schedules.* Busy healthcare executives should recognize that board members too are very busy. Trustees are devoting their precious time to serve the organization, and the time they spend in board meetings is time taken away from their families and careers. CEOs should ensure that all meetings start on time and are run as efficiently as possible.

- *Manage controversy.* Controversial issues can sometimes arise unexpectedly during the course of a board meeting. Ideally, discussion on these topics should be postponed until later to allow for consensus building and thorough preparation. However, controversial issues cannot be put off forever, and CEOs should work with trustees to place any such issues on a future agenda so that a thoughtful and informed dialogue can take place.

- *Understand board members' community roles.* Trustees will likely have other community activities and organizations that they favor. The hospital—and the CEO personally—should make a point to support those organizations as well.

Manage the Board Wisely

The most successful CEOs have developed tactics to manage the board to help accomplish the daily work of the organization and to advance the overall strategic plan. They ensure that trustees are well informed and knowledgeable of the board's oversight role, but they also work diplomatically to keep the board from micromanaging details that should be the responsibility of the executive team. The following actions can help maintain this delicate balance of power:

- *Manage the flow of information.* Healthcare trustees are often successful leaders in their own right, and they can rapidly assess the elements of a situation and come to recommendations and conclusions. When presenting issues or proposals to the board, the CEO should use an executive summary format to glean the key points and to preserve time for discussion. Distributing information ahead of formal meetings—allowing trustees to read the materials in advance—can be helpful, particularly for complicated topics. Doing so can ensure that the meeting itself is focused on thoughtful dialogue rather than on the recounting of facts that could have been read in a report.

- *Learn the board's preference for detail.* This action may seem simplistic, but CEOs must gauge and measure the board's preference for information. Some boards prefer quantity, whereas others prefer brief summaries. The type and quality of information desired may also change as a board's leadership changes. Our counsel is simple: Test the waters occasionally, and ask if the board members feel they are getting the proper quality and quantity of information.

- *Run the hospital well.* The best way to manage a board is to do a great job managing the organization. If trustees see that you and your leadership team are competent and are performing well on key metrics, they will develop a level of trust that will facilitate effective interactions in the future.

- *Be positive about the organization's past leadership.* Executives should never cast a negative light on their predecessors or on their predecessors' leadership actions. Doing so not only is bad form, but it also risks stirring feelings of animosity in cases where current trustees have personal relationships with former executives.

- *Coordinate formal communications.* The CEO must be the sole channel through which all formal board documents, reports, agendas, and meeting appointments pass between the organization and the board. Multiple channels can lead to multiple sources of "truth"—which can result in confusion, conflict, and unnecessary duplication of work.

Regularly Review Board Functionality

Just as CEOs conduct regular performance appraisals for members of the leadership team, they should also have a formal mechanism for evaluating the effectiveness of each individual trustee and the performance of the board overall. Most organizations conduct an annual survey of each board member that generates feedback about the trustees' sense of being well prepared to conduct their duties, areas in which the executive team can improve, and suggestions of how communication or board meetings can be enhanced.

Increasingly, CEOs are asked to provide their opinions on the value that each trustee brings to the organization. The results of these surveys are reviewed between the CEO and the board chair in an effort to improve the quality of the board over time. A key decision point when contemplating a trustee evaluation process is determining who will be responsible for providing feedback to the trustees about their individual assessments. Choosing the right person or group to act on the evaluation is as important a decision as whether to perform the evaluation at all. Many organizations have the board chairperson discuss the results with board members, whereas other organizations rely on an influential peer director or a formal committee of the board to hold these sometimes-sensitive discussions.

SUMMARY

Working with the board is often more of an art than a science, and the art usually requires the application of common sense, communication skills, and relationship building. The burden placed on modern healthcare trustees is tremendous, and membership on a board can expose community volunteers to great legal and reputational damage if issues arise. Because trustees are willing to accept this risk in an effort to improve the healthcare delivery system in their community, each and every board member should be shown the utmost respect. Executive teams can manifest this respect by investing in board education to help prepare trustees for their roles, by communicating with trustees effectively and completely, and by providing them with regular feedback to help them grow in their roles as directors. This investment of time and energy will not only result in a more competent and effective board; it will also facilitate the organization's achievement of strategic goals.

REFLECTIVE QUESTIONS

1. What does the orientation process look like for new board members in your organization? How could it be enhanced?

2. What are some of the new quality and outcomes programs that have come about as a result of the Affordable Care Act? What would be the role of your organization's board in overseeing these programs?

RESOURCES AND EXERCISES FOR LEADERSHIP DEVELOPMENT

1. To gain a better understanding of boards, consult the following books:

Biggs, E. L. 2011. *Healthcare Governance: A Guide for Effective Boards*, 2nd ed. Chicago: Health Administration Press.

Carver, J. 2006. *Boards That Make a Difference: A New Design for Leadership in Nonprofit and Public Organizations*, 3rd ed. San Francisco: Jossey-Bass.

2. There is no better way to learn about boards than to become a board member. Leaders should give serious consideration to joining the board of a local not-for-profit organization. The experience, as well as the service provided, can greatly enrich any healthcare leader's life.

3. Review *A Self-Assessment Guide for Health Care Organizations*, by the International Finance Corporation (www.ifc.org/wps/wcm/connect/509355004970c21ca215f23 36b93d75f/IFCSelfAssessGuide.pdf?MOD=AJPERES).

REFERENCES

American College of Healthcare Executives. 2015. "Hospital CEO Turnover 1981–2015." Published March 5. www.ache.org/pubs /research/ceoturnover.cfm.

Davidson, P. S., and T. R. Murdock. 2013. "Legal Duties and Avoiding Liability: A Nonprofit Board Member Primer." *Trustee*. Published June 10. www.trusteemag.com/display/TRU-news-article .dhtml?dcrPath=/templatedata/HF_Common/NewsArticle /data/TRU/WebExclusives/2013/WebExclusive0613legalduties.

National Quality Forum. 2004. *Hospital Governing Boards and Quality of Care: A Call to Responsibility*. Institute for Healthcare Improvement. Accessed February 15, 2015. www.ihi.org /resources/Pages/Publications/HospitalGoverningBoardsand QualityofCareACalltoResponsibility.aspx.

CHAPTER 9

Human Resources

Always recognize that human individuals are ends, and do not use them as means to your end.

—Immanuel Kant

Guide to Reader

Savvy leaders will attest to the fact that effective "people" strategies can be the difference between career-ending falls and great organizational triumphs. In regard to protocols, human resources is the area where the most eyes will be watching, the most ears will be hearing, and the most judgments will be made. Though serious ethical missteps might rank as the most costly career blunders, slip-ups with people most certainly follow closely.

The Worst-Kept Secret

The CEO of a well-known integrated healthcare system had become increasingly dissatisfied with the performance of the senior vice president (SVP) of ambulatory services, the executive team member responsible for the planning and execution of the organization's aggressive outpatient strategy. From an objective standpoint, the ambulatory division had enjoyed great success under this executive's leadership, opening 10 new outpatient centers in key markets over the past 24 months, each exceeding both budget and volume expectations. The SVP was also well respected by his peers and universally acknowledged (even by the CEO) to be a talented leader with superb strategic, analytical, and operations expertise. The issues that had arisen between the CEO and the ambulatory executive were more related to a difference in leadership and communication styles. Moreover, the CEO perceived that the SVP was too quick to challenge the CEO's ideas and did not show him the appropriate amount of deference.

Rather than discuss these concerns directly with the SVP to develop mutually acceptable ground rules that might improve their working relationship, the CEO made the decision that the executive was a bad "fit" with the leadership team and needed to be removed. He began voicing his displeasure in private meetings with other members of the executive team and spoke of his plans to dismiss the SVP. The ambulatory SVP, a well-liked member of the executive team, eventually was made aware of the CEO's intentions by his peer executives, who felt it was unfair that he could lose his job over a personality conflict.

(continued)

(continued from previous page)

Over the next several weeks, the ambulatory executive continued to perform his job duties in a professional manner, but he also began interviewing for a similar role with the organization's chief competitor in the market. By the time the CEO scheduled a meeting to formally terminate the executive, he was in for a shock: The SVP not only was aware of the CEO's intentions but also had already agreed to join their competitor, with several members of the organization's ambulatory division staff committed to follow him. In a period of two years, this executive led his new organization to become the market leader in outpatient services, outpacing his prior employer by a wide margin.

Be mindful: No task is more challenging, or more rewarding, than that of managing people. Remember that this role is a privilege and that your employees have entrusted you with their professional destiny. As a leader, you must earn that trust every day by managing in an ethical manner.

HUMAN RESOURCES AS A STRATEGIC PARTNER

Historically, the role of the CEO in healthcare has focused largely on strategic planning and growth functions; meanwhile, the responsibility for personnel management has often been relegated to a human resources (HR) executive with a relatively marginal role within the leadership team. In recent years, however, economic troubles and legislative changes have brought workforce management issues to the forefront, requiring a more effective partnership between the CEO and the chief HR officer. To be flexible and efficient in times of change, leadership teams must be adept at a variety of challenging workforce initiatives, including broad-based talent management, efforts to reduce labor costs, programs to raise staff competency levels, and promotion of a culture that fosters high morale and employee engagement.

In a service industry such as healthcare, salaries and benefit costs are by far the largest component of operating expenses. Workforce management thus has a direct impact on the achievement of profitability objectives, particularly in light of shrinking reimbursement. In addition, healthcare in recent years has become increasingly transparent, with unified core-measure quality data nationally published and best-practice sharing commonplace. With this transparency, operational processes can easily be replicated across organizations; as a result, the only true sustainable competitive advantage an organization can enjoy is the quality of its workforce.

These dynamics have led senior leaders to take a much more active role in the development and execution of "people" strategies for their organizations and to raise workforce management to a higher level of strategic focus. In light of this elevation, the role of the chief human resources officer must change: Rather than serving simply as a content expert, the HR officer should lead as a strategic executive partner to the CEO and the senior leadership team. However, as shown in Exhibit 9.1, this evolution is still a work in progress for many organizations, especially as it pertains to human resources involvement in the strategic planning process.

EXHIBIT 9.1: Human Resources Involvement in Strategic Planning
- 33 percent of HR executives say they are "on the sidelines" during the planning process.
- 22 percent of senior HR executives indicate that they are consulted during the planning process but are below the executive team level.
- Only 19 percent of senior HR executives consider themselves part of the executive team.
- 10 percent of HR executives are completely excluded from growth planning.

Source: Human Resource Planning Society (2009).

A strategic disconnect between the senior leadership team and the "people" function of the organization can lead to significant issues in translating strategy into action. In today's environment, leaders in healthcare must assume human resources roles for their areas of responsibility, with an eye toward retention, accountability, motivation, efficiency, competency, and succession planning. All leaders must increase their formal knowledge of human resources competencies and apply this knowledge in their daily work of executing the organization's strategic objectives. Likewise, HR leaders must strengthen their knowledge of the business and develop people strategies that support the overarching goals of the organization. Even more important than content knowledge, however, is the need for executive leaders to adjudicate decisions related to workforce management in an appropriately sensitive manner.

EFFECTIVE HUMAN RESOURCES MANAGEMENT

Ethics and sensitivity have numerous well-known implications for a healthcare organization and the community it serves. Often overlooked, however, are the ethical and emotional implications of the human resources decisions made by healthcare executives. An executive's burden of leadership includes true responsibility for each employee's livelihood, and every human resources decision has a direct effect on the staff. Within the confines of the executive suite, some daily decisions may seem to go unseen; in reality, however, employees watch and remember all executive decisions, even those decisions that do not pertain to them directly. If the decisions are poorly informed, do not demonstrate appropriate cultural sensitivity, or, in extreme cases, are unethical or illegal, they become part of the organizational lore for years to come, significantly damaging the credibility of the leadership team. The risk of these missteps is greatest in human resources situations where emotions naturally run high, such as employee terminations or reductions in force. Rarely will an executive knowingly execute an unethical or illegal decision; however, issues can quickly arise if a leader is poorly informed, does not fully understand the culture, or is ignorant of applicable laws and policies. Therefore, leaders at all levels should have a framework for developing human resources content knowledge and a method for adjudicating sensitive decisions on people management. The following protocol, summarized in Exhibit 9.2, aims to assist in this regard.

EXHIBIT 9.2: Protocol for Human Resources Management

The following framework can facilitate ethical and strategic human resources management:

1. Know the laws and regulations.
2. Make ethical human resources decisions.
3. Treat others with respect.
4. Understand nuances of compensation and benefits.
5. Invest in developing talent.
6. Develop metrics of effectiveness for the human resources function.

Know the Laws and Regulations

Unless leaders have advanced in their careers along a human resources track, they likely develop their knowledge of labor and employment law based on trial and error and some formal education from graduate school (which might be out of date). Though CEOs and other leaders need not be experts in all employment matters (they can rely on the HR executive for comprehensive expertise), a true strategic "people" focus requires at least a working understanding of the most important human resources laws and policies. The following actions can assist in developing a broader understanding of HR regulations:

- *Build personal regulatory knowledge.* Either through a formal continuing-education process or through mentoring with a human resources expert, leaders should develop their knowledge of basic labor laws and the way those laws are applied in the healthcare environment. They should be familiar with regulations related to fair labor standards, discrimination, hostile work environments, sexual harassment, and collective bargaining and unionization. Taking the time to know and understand these laws does not ensure that leaders will always make ethical decisions, but it does help provide insight into their ethical intent. Leaders should consider the meaning and spirit behind the laws when formulating human resources policy.

- *Understand all human resources policies.* Leaders should possess a firm understanding of organizational policies and procedures pertaining to people management. Because regulations vary from state to state (e.g., different "at will" employment practices), leaders should not assume that policies in an organization they have newly joined will be the same as those of their prior organization. Senior leaders must ensure not only that personnel policies follow the applicable laws but also that the associated procedures have a well-thought-out rationale. The rationale should be clearly stated within the policies and should set the guidelines under which the policies are enforced.

- *Establish a system of due process for employees.* A system of due process provides an opportunity for employees to question the decisions of an organization and helps ensure that just and ethical decisions are reached. The due process system should be clearly articulated in policy, and all employees should be educated on their right to seek resolution of concerns through appropriate channels. Leaders should make due process much more than just a means to resolve conflict; it should be a corporate attitude that proves to the staff that the organization has a sincere interest in employees and their concerns. An engaged and open culture fosters more effective leadership decisions on personnel matters, and it reduces the need for employees to seek resolution through external agencies and lawsuits.

Make Ethical Human Resources Decisions

Of all the decisions leaders make, none have a greater impact on the lives of employees and the culture of the organization than decisions related to human resources. Terminating employees, managing layoffs, counseling low performers, and deciding whom to hire are key responsibilities of leadership roles, and the manner in which leaders execute these decisions has a dramatic impact on how they are perceived by frontline employees. Such decisions must be carried out in a rational, ethical manner, with the utmost respect and dignity provided to employees. The following actions can assist leaders in managing difficult decisions:

- *Be as quantitative as possible.* The changing healthcare environment, shifting reimbursement patterns, and shrinking margins have led to pervasive reductions in force as organizations try to rightsize their fixed-cost infrastructure for a future with less inpatient utilization. Of course, no employees want to be told that they are going to lose their jobs. However, if leaders use objective metrics and are transparent with their thought processes, staff are more likely to perceive a sense of fairness relating to such decisions. One metric that executives can use to guide decisions involving labor costs is the *labor cost revenue percentage*—that is, the expenses associated with staff as a percentage of revenues (see Exhibit 9.3). Most organizations spend from 22 to 35 cents in labor for every dollar of revenue. The senior leadership team should set a goal for this metric that encourages efficiency and ensures

EXHIBIT 9.3: Labor Cost Revenue Percentage

$$\text{Labor Cost Revenue Percentage} = \frac{\text{Compensation + Benefits Cost}}{\text{Annual Revenues}} \times 100$$

the ongoing financial viability of the organization (without sacrificing clinical safety).

- *Be as objective as possible.* Objectivity suggests such concepts as fairness, balance, and good judgment. However, these concepts have different meanings to different people, so true objectivity is difficult to put into practice. Leaders who are adept at being objective are ones who listen intently without interrupting, realize that every situation has some uniqueness within it, and strive to seek out facts when confronted with problems laden with emotion. The field of human resources is filled with laws, rules, and regulations dealing with fairness and objectivity, but leaders should seek to reflect those principles beyond just the written law. Exhibit 9.4 provides a list of characteristics of objective leadership.

EXHIBIT 9.4: What Makes a Leader Objective?
- Ability and willingness to step back and see things from more than just one's own personal viewpoint
- Ability and willingness to recognize and manage biases, prejudices, and preconceived notions
- Ability and willingness to remain personally neutral and allow facts to drive decision making
- Ability and willingness to manage emotion and stress and see through the fog of passion

- *Consider the effects of all decisions, especially when the decisions involve termination.* If a human resources decision involves termination—known by some as "economic capital punishment"—feelings and egos will inevitably be hurt in the process. Although some struggling employees may initially feel relieved when they are terminated, the process is disheartening to everyone involved. Many organizations have a rule that forbids terminating any employee without the approval of the chief HR officer, the CEO, or both. This system of checks and balances helps ensure fairness and consistency in the application of progressive discipline and termination. It also allows someone other than the immediate supervisor to review the facts of each case and make sure that personal biases do not cloud objective judgment. Ideally, all ethical dimensions will be considered, and the fairness of the decision will be ensured. The decision to terminate an employee should be considered a last resort, and all applicable procedures related to progressive discipline must be closely followed. All appropriate evidence should be collected prior to the termination meeting, and the discussion should be held by the leader who made the decision to terminate. The discussion should not be delegated.

- *Evaluate the end result first.* Senior leaders often review human resources decisions recommended by lower-level managers. When assessing such decisions, the leaders should always determine the cost and risk of a decision relative to its potential benefit. Some decisions involving employees may be driven by a supervisor's ego or desire for power, and they may result in no demonstrable benefit to the organization. If no good will result from the decision, or if it is not backed by objective data, the decision should not stand.

- *Evaluate who will benefit the most.* In all human resources decisions, the leader should consider how to best maintain a balance between what is needed by the organization and what is needed by the employee. Remember that the leader's ultimate responsibility is to be a fiduciary of the organization as a whole; this responsibility should always be the determining factor when difficult decisions need to be made.

Treat Others with Respect

Leaders have little difficulty treating employees with respect during times of plenty, but when challenging employee matters arise, common courtesy sometimes becomes an afterthought. Leaders can demonstrate respect by remaining consistent in their actions and following some simple guidelines:

- *Develop and follow a human resources philosophy.* Leaders should institute and live by a human resources philosophy or values statement on both individual and corporate levels. This document should be highly visible in the organization and serve as a "contract" with employees that states how they can expect to be treated. Exhibit 9.5 provides an example of a corporate human resources philosophy statement.
- *Treat employees with the same amount of respect when you terminate their employment as you did when you hired them.* Under certain circumstances, the termination of an employee is unavoidable. In these instances, the employee should be treated with the utmost respect during the process of separating from the organization. Prior to termination, the employee should receive appropriate warnings and performance feedback in line with the

organization's progressive discipline policy. The ultimate communication of termination should not come as a surprise to the employee. Consider legal ramifications and discuss the events with human resources and potentially legal counsel, particularly if the employee is a manager or in a protected legal classification. Develop a separation agreement and release-of-liability form for the employee to sign.

On the day of the formal termination, be on time to the meeting and get to the point quickly. Be kind in the choice of language but firm in the delivery of the message. Do not get into a debate around the decision to terminate—the time for negotiations about continued employment should be over. Discuss plans for the announcement of the termination for internal staff and external releases (if appropriate). Allowing the employee some input into the communication process can provide a semblance of control in a difficult situation. Depending on tenure and circumstances, consider using outplacement services to help the employee find his next role. Offering these services demonstrates respect and a true desire to assist the employee to be successful even if he was the wrong fit for your organization.

Understand the Nuances of Compensation and Benefits

Many studies on organizational behavior have indicated that salary and benefits alone are not a driver of long-term employee motivation; nonetheless, the lack of competitive compensation can still place an organization at a competitive disadvantage in recruiting and retaining talent. Leaders must balance the need for efficient operations and expense control with the need to keep salary and benefits at a level that will keep staff engaged. The following ideas may assist in this regard:

- *Understand the market.* Remaining competitive from a salary standpoint is a top concern for hiring managers, as it can directly correlate with the ability to attract and retain top talent in the labor market. The aim is to find a pay level that makes your organization an employer of choice, while achieving that status at the lowest possible cost. Striking this balance requires that organizations conduct market research to understand the pay practices of other employers and think creatively to devise competitive compensation packages that do not add too much cost.

    Once salary ranges for the market have been identified, leaders must benchmark individual employees' salaries relative to the overall range. Doing so helps reward and retain top performers and ensures that employees do not fall behind the market. One key metric that can assist in this regard is the *compa-ratio*, which divides an employee's salary by the median of the salary range for her position (see Exhibit 9.6). A compa-ratio of 1.00 means that the employee is paid at the median of the range. Employees who are paid at a compa-ratio below 1.00 are at risk of falling behind the market (particularly if they are experienced or tenured), which may lead to job dissatisfaction and turnover.

EXHIBIT 9.6: Compa-ratio
Compa-ratio = Employee's Salary / Midpoint of Salary Range

- *Use benefits strategically.* One way of creating a competitive compensation strategy without overpaying from a pure salary standpoint is to enhance the fringe benefits for employees in the organization. An aggressive employer match in a retirement plan or a lower deductible for health benefits, for instance, can be key decision-making factors for employees, particularly in markets with pay parity. Of course, benefits also come at a cost, and this cost needs to be managed to a reasonable level. A key management metric in this area is *benefits cost per employee*, calculated by dividing total benefits costs by the total number of employees (see Exhibit 9.7). Most organizations trend around 20–35 percent in this ratio. Executives should investigate causes of benefit-cost "creep" that might be indicative of changes in employee behavior (e.g., greater participation in retirement plans, increased use of health benefits).

EXHIBIT 9.7: Benefits Cost per Employee
Benefits Cost per Employee = Total Benefits Costs / Number of Employees

---

Invest in Developing Talent

Most companies in general business discovered long ago that their people are their most precious commodity and that investment in growing talent within the organization brings a tremendous return over time. According to a survey, nearly 95 percent of *Fortune* 500 companies reported having a structured employee development program in place; however, only 25 percent of hospital CEOs responded similarly (Lee and Herring 2009). In a dynamic environment such as healthcare, development of a capable and well-trained workforce creates a key strategic advantage because it enables an organization to respond to changes in the market more quickly. In addition, leadership development and succession planning provide upward mobility for talented staff members and ensure continuity of strategy in the event that turnover occurs in key positions. Historically, education programs in healthcare environments have focused on building the clinical skills of caregivers, and this focus will remain important in the future. However, competencies around quality, regulatory compliance, and patient satisfaction will be equally critical for success and are not as widely understood among frontline staff. CEOs must recognize that they are in the people-development business: They should work with their HR executive partners to develop a staff development plan that will create skills in the employee base to support organizational strategic objectives.

Develop Metrics of Effectiveness for the Human Resources Function

As leaders at all levels in healthcare place greater strategic focus on people management, their human resources partners should expect to be held accountable for providing appropriate levels of service to internal customers in the organization. Just as a chief nursing officer is expected to manage patient care units at staffing levels in line with nurse-to-patient ratios based on acuity, the performance of a human resources department should be tracked and measured against established metrics of success. Staff turnover, as a general rule, has a negative impact on healthcare organizations because it can disrupt the care team, lower morale, and necessitate costly recruitment efforts. As a result, it typically is the first HR metric to be tracked. Leaders should evaluate the turnover in their areas of responsibility and watch for increasing resignations and other worrisome trends; such trends may be indicative of underlying issues (e.g., supervisory concerns, poor workplace conditions) that need to be addressed. One easy way to track turnover is to calculate the *monthly turnover metric*, by dividing the number of people who left the company in the past month by the total number of employees (see Exhibit 9.8). In smaller organizations, or at the departmental level, turnover should be tracked on a daily basis, with exit interviews conducted for each voluntary turnover to determine what issues need to be addressed to enhance employee retention.

EXHIBIT 9.8: Monthly Turnover
Monthly Turnover = Employees Separated / Number of Employees × 100

Even with an organization's best efforts to avoid turnover, sometimes family or environmental conditions make the loss of key staff members inevitable. When turnover does occur, leaders should hold their human resources partners accountable for filling vacancies in a timely and efficient fashion. Executives can track this process by quantifying the number of days from the time of turnover to the time the position is filled, as well as by monitoring the overall *cost per hire*. The latter is a key metric that can be calculated by dividing the overall recruitment costs by the total number of new hires (see Exhibit 9.9).

SUMMARY

The development of a people-focused culture requires the active attention of all leaders within the organization; it can no longer be solely the responsibility of the human resources function. Operational leaders must understand the staff competencies required to achieve strategic goals, and HR executives must be accountable for delivering the services required for the organization to be successful. In an environment that is becoming increasingly competitive for top talent, healthcare leaders should look to enhance their own competencies in building and sustaining a culture that is fair, ethical, and supportive to employees; such leaders will differentiate themselves in the minds of staff and help their organization become an employer of choice.

GUEST COMMENTARY: BILL MCLEAN

After approximately 30 years in the healthcare industry and human resources field, I have experienced or observed enough human behavior in the workplace to come to some conclusions.

First, according to a sermon I heard about 20 years ago—and I have since seen literature supporting this point—the number-one human need is to feel appreciated. If leaders would take this one little premise seriously, most other management practices would fall into place naturally.

(continued)

(continued from previous page)

Second, leaders are like parents. Your employees, like children, observe the way you behave and treat people far more closely than they listen to your words.

Third, the authors state that the only true sustainable competitive advantage a healthcare organization can enjoy is the quality of its workforce. I have always preached that our only sustainable advantage is the ability to leverage our people, processes, and technology—and with nearly 60 percent of our expenses wrapped up in labor, paying attention to our people is the number-one priority.

Fourth, to be a good leader, you need to know the rules and regulations of how to legally deal with your people. However, that information serves merely as a guide. I have always been blessed with logical and fair-minded legal counsel. We strive to make good and fair business decisions first, and *then* we look back to make sure we have solid legal footing—not the other way around. This approach has kept us true to the intent of taking care of people.

Fifth, we believe healthcare is a ministry, but we also recognize that it is big business. Leaders have many metrics to follow, and they are all important. However, one larger concept that often is not followed is that all leaders should run their part of the business as though they owned the entire enterprise. They should imagine that they are the singular owner of the whole operation and that leadership of the organization represents their only job and only source of income. Leaders would then create metrics they would follow religiously.

(continued)

(continued from previous page)

Finally, many years ago there was a book by Robert Fulghum titled *All I Really Need to Know I Learned in Kindergarten* (Villard, 1988). The book offers so many accurate pointers that it should be required reading. The message comes down to caring about people. Hire the best, and help them become the best they can become. In the end, you will retain the ones you want because they will recognize the kind of employer you are. It almost seems too easy, but this is what a truly great leader does.

Bill McLean
Senior Vice President, Human Resources
Avera Health
Sioux Falls, South Dakota

REFLECTIVE QUESTIONS

1. Review the human resources and employment policies in your organization. Are the procedures clearly written? How could they be enhanced?

2. Review the employee termination story in the vignette at the beginning of this chapter. What could the CEO have done differently to create a better outcome?

3. Answer this question honestly: Do you truly believe that people are the greatest asset of an organization?

RESOURCES AND EXERCISES FOR LEADERSHIP DEVELOPMENT

1. Research the concept of "advocacy" and discuss what advocacy means with a human resources expert.

2. One of the downfalls of many HR leaders is a lack of perceptual objectivity, and operations managers often feel HR leaders are oblivious to their needs as managers. Discuss with several HR leaders (a) how they approach problem situations with a clear perception of organizational and political realities and (b) how they stay sensitive to the operating needs of the organization.

3. Readers seeking more in-depth information on human resources metrics should consult the following books:

> Fitz-enz, J. 2010. *The New HR Analytics: Predicting the Economic Value of Your Company's Human Capital Investments.* New York: AMACOM.

> Pease, G., B. Byerly, and J. Fitz-enz. 2012. *Human Capital Analytics: How to Harness the Potential of Your Organization's Greatest Asset.* Hoboken, NJ: Wiley.

4. David Ulrich provides a contemporary view of the various roles that human resources plays in an organization. Consider the model shown on the next page and describe how it affects leaders in different positions in an organization.

Practical Application of Human Resources Roles
STRATEGIC (LONG-TERM)

<table>
<tr><td valign="top" rowspan="2">PROCESS</td><td valign="top">

Customer need: Effective business and HR strategies

Ownership: 85% line, 15% HR

HR function: Alignment

Role: Strategic HR leadership

Competencies:

- Business knowledge
- HR strategy formulation
- Influencing skills

HR needs to be well-versed in the business to ensure that they are supporting the key strategies.

</td><td valign="top">

Customer need: Organizational effectiveness

Ownership: 75% line, 25% HR

HR function: Change management

Role: Change agent

Competencies:

- Change management skills
- Consulting/facilitation/ coaching
- Systems analysis skills

HR must have expertise in change management and serve as the in-house resources to manage change.

</td><td valign="top" rowspan="2">PEOPLE</td></tr>
<tr><td valign="top">

Customer need: High-touch, high-value administrative processes; efficiency; records; information

Ownership: 25% line, 75% HR

HR function: Services / record keeping

Role: Function manager

Competencies:

- Content knowledge
- Process improvement
- Information from HRIS
- Customer relations
- Service-needs assessment

HR must run an efficient department focused on service to line managers, helping to make the HR components of their jobs more effective and ensure compliance in HR legal issues.

</td><td valign="top">

Customer need: Employee commitment

Ownership: 75% line, 25% HR

HR function: Employee relations

Role: Employee sponsor/ advocate

Competencies:

- Work environment assessment
- Management / employee development
- Performance management
- Reward and recognition

HR must develop programs that ensure fairness for employees, open communication lines, and due process provisions.

</td></tr>
</table>

OPERATIONAL (DAY-TO-DAY)

Source: Reprinted with permission from Ulrich (1996).

REFERENCES

Human Resources Planning Society. 2009. *HR's Role in Strategic Planning.* New York: Human Resources Planning Society.

Lee, B. D., and J. W. Herring. 2009. *Growing Leaders in Healthcare: Lessons from the Corporate World.* Chicago: Health Administration Press.

Ulrich, D. 1996. *Human Resource Champions: The Next Agenda for Adding Value and Delivering Results.* Boston: Harvard Business School Press.

CHAPTER 10

Communications, Technology, and Social Media

Regardless of the changes in technology, the market for well-crafted messages will always have an audience.

—Steve Burnett

Guide to Reader

Communication—listening and talking, holding meetings, sending e-mails, presenting PowerPoints, persuading and directing others, and participating in LinkedIn, Facebook, Twitter, and other social media. All these actions—and many more—come to mind when one thinks of leadership. It can be said that communication is the lifeblood of leadership; without it, leadership dies. Communication touches every aspect of leadership, from crafting vision to executing plans to leading change. Yet at the same time, it can be the foundation for the most severe stumbles that leaders suffer.

The Merger That Wasn't

In anticipation of significant changes in the postreform era, the leaders of two nonprofit healthcare delivery systems that had historically been competitors decided that their greatest chance for success would be to build scale and negotiating power through a merger into a single network. The respective CEOs and board members for the organizations met several times over the course of a year to map out the parameters of the deal. After much discussion, they decided that the larger of the two systems would become the dominant brand and that the CEO of that organization would be the leader of the new, merged entity. The CEO of the smaller organization would stay on as system COO, and the boards would be merged into a unified structure, with the most senior members placed on the system board and the more junior members serving on various functional committees. A letter of intent was signed to move forward with the initiative, and both CEOs began communicating the plan to their leadership teams and employees.

Both CEOs carefully crafted messages about the deal structure and attempted to convey their excitement around the prospect of moving forward together. The messages, however, failed to have the desired effect. Having been so deeply involved in the merger discussions over the past year, the CEOs fully understood the strategic rationale behind the merger, and they assumed their employees would understand as well. They did not spend much time explaining the implications of the significant changes in the healthcare environment, the effects of those changes on the local market, and the benefits of building scale both from the standpoint of improving negotiating position and

(continued)

(continued from previous page)

influencing population health. As a result, the message around merging with an organization that had been the "enemy" seemed confusing and counterintuitive to employees. The CEOs also began an e-mail campaign to inform employees about the timeline of the merger process. However, the messages came across as tactical, did not provide sufficient information about the benefits of the proposed structure, and failed to assuage real fears about job loss in the merger process.

Employees from both organizations launched campaigns on social media to rally their peers, former patients, and community members to keep the hospitals separate. The campaigns emphasized concerns about losing the "unique culture" that each organization had built and how the merger might negatively affect the care provided to patients within their communities. The efforts exerted a great deal of pressure on the board members. The organizations made subsequent attempts to more effectively communicate the benefits of the merger and turn the tide of public opinion, but ultimately the organizations bowed to the pressure and agreed not to merge. Less than two years later, the organizations were purchased by separate investor-owned hospital-operating companies. They remain fierce competitors.

Be mindful: Because leaders often deal with numerous demands at once, employees typically form impressions of them through a series of brief interactions over time. Being thoughtful about each of these interactions can help ensure that the staff has a positive mental image of you as their leader and of the decisions you make. Problems with culture and poor communication can derail even the most well-thought-out strategies.

THE IMPORTANCE OF COMMUNICATION

In the dynamic and complex environment of a healthcare organization, clinicians regularly make decisions that have a dramatic impact—positive or negative—on the lives of the patients being served. Likewise, healthcare leaders frequently make decisions that have a dramatic impact on the overall health and sustainability of the organization. When a major decision is made, leaders rely on frontline staff to understand the rationale for the decision and to execute the decision in a manner that will move the organization toward its goal. Communication is critically important in garnering staff support, and it can make the difference between success and failure for otherwise talented executives.

Communication is essential for effective functioning in every part of a healthcare organization. Staff can receive broad direction from organizational documents such as a strategic plan, but leaders within the organization have the responsibility to translate these goals into actions that are understood and endorsed by the front line. Executives who lack proper communication skills will struggle to gain support and often can create animosity inadvertently because of poorly worded or ambiguous directions.

Historically, leaders were judged on their ability to produce results and on the "hard skills" of business planning and financial management. In recent years, however, organizations have become increasingly aware that excellent performance can be better sustained with an additional focus on the "soft skills" of communication, humility, and respect. Today, executives are judged not only on the results they achieve but also on the manner in which they achieve them. A survey of top US executives (summarized in Exhibit 10.1) found that leadership skills such as integrity and communication were rated as "extremely important" to overall organizational success by more than 90 percent of the senior leaders polled (Robles 2012).

EXHIBIT 10.1: Leadership Attributes and the Percentage of Executives Rating Them "Extremely Important"

- Integrity: 93%
- Communication: 91%
- Courtesy: 85%
- Responsibility: 72%
- Interpersonal skills: 61%
- Positive attitude: 47%
- Teamwork: 43%
- Flexibility: 42%
- Work ethic: 36%

Source: Robles (2012).

Effective communication takes many forms—especially in today's environment, where modern communications systems and approaches all present different benefits, appropriate uses, and challenges. Advances in technology have allowed for the proliferation of information on a scale and speed that were unthinkable a generation ago. Executives today must have the ability to craft effective messages, to understand the methods for broadcasting messages, to know how to manage multiple information systems, and to determine which methods are most appropriate for specific situations. In this chapter, we share protocols for enhancing your interactions—whether formal interactions in the boardroom, informal ones in a hallway, or those on paper, in e-mail, or over social media.

EFFECTIVE VERBAL COMMUNICATION

Verbal, or spoken, communication is the most direct and intimate form of communication. Most experts agree that it is typically the most effective. Verbal communication reveals emotion—passion, joy, anger, stress, concern, or excitement—of both the communicator and the receiver(s) of the communication. It is unfettered and personal, and its impact is observable, memorable, and influential. A leader's approach to verbal communication will vary depending on the setting (informal chat versus formal presentation), audience (employee forum versus board meeting), and subject (celebrating excellent results versus communicating a layoff); thus the message must be crafted to meet the specific needs of the situation. Carefully crafting the message greatly enhances the likelihood that the communication will achieve its desired result. What does all this mean? Simply this: The preparation for communication requires forethought, planning, agility, sensitivity, and caution. The following protocol, summarized in Exhibit 10.2, can assist in this regard.

EXHIBIT 10.2: Protocol for Effective Verbal Communication

The following framework can assist in crafting effective verbal messages:
1. Practice dialogue, not monologue.
2. Actively listen.
3. Be concise.
4. Be aware of nonverbal messages.
5. Prepare, prepare, prepare.

Practice Dialogue, Not Monologue

Getting a point across hinges on a two-way interaction, especially in the communication of a complex rationale or instruction. Open exchange and feedback are important in ensuring that both parties understand and agree with the direction being taken. Too often, however, time constraints and busy schedules relegate executives to an "information sharing" mode, in which they pontificate in individual and group settings without giving others a chance to respond. Once these patterns have been established, subordinates often become too intimidated to ask for clarification and may interpret messages incorrectly. The following steps can help create an atmosphere that encourages interactive dialogue:

- Take a deep breath and be deliberate in the delivery of your message to avoid seeming rushed.
- Pause frequently to give staff the time to ask clarifying questions.
- Ask staff to repeat the message in their own words to ensure understanding.
- Follow up through employee rounding to reinforce the key messages and obtain feedback.
- Follow up with a written summary or e-mail.

Actively Listen

Senior leaders often approach personal interactions with a goal of solving problems, rather than seeking feedback and truly listening to the needs and viewpoints of those with whom they communicate. This tendency can lead not only to frustration and misunderstanding but also to wasted efforts by executives who have not taken the time to discern the key issues important to the staff. Listening to what someone has to say is a sign of respect, and it can promote a culture of openness if leaders act on the feedback that they receive. In group and individual interactions, remember the adage: "You have two ears and one mouth; therefore listen twice as much as you speak."

Be Concise

Executives should strive to craft verbal communication that is simple, can be delivered in a short amount of time, touches on all the salient points of the strategic message, and allows an opportunity for interactive discussion. When rounding in the organization, leaders should have a weekly list of five key initiatives or issues that they want to reinforce with the staff, and they should use this list as a basis for interactions with the units. Leaders should also ask direct reports to create their own weekly "Friday Five" lists that they share with their staffs. The short lists prepared by direct reports can also help leaders keep abreast of the important issues in their areas of responsibility. Exhibit 10.3 offers additional pointers for being succinct in your communication.

Be Aware of Nonverbal Messages

Leaders should manage their nonverbal communication as carefully as they manage their words. Even seemingly insignificant details—for instance, staying behind your desk when someone enters your office instead of coming around to meet him—have potential to offend people with whom you interact. Eye contact, facial expressions, and body language indicate a person's mind-set and often can send a more powerful message than what is being spoken. Appropriate nonverbal cues can be the difference between an employee's perception of interest or distraction, emotion or lack of it, and attention or disregard. Leaders should maintain appropriate personal space, consistent eye contact, and open and approachable body language. Their facial expressions should express that they have heard and understood what employees have shared.

EXHIBIT 10.3: Want to Be More Succinct?
- Use fewer words.
- Use words with clarity.
- Use simple words.
- Use fewer adjectives.
- Get to the point.
- Repeat your key message.
- Think: "bumper sticker."

Prepare, Prepare, Prepare

In presentations and formal communications, preparation—both internal and external—is key to success. Internal preparation demands that the speaker learn and understand the specific material and overall subject matter to be discussed. External preparation involves the specific details of the presentation, such as the supporting slide deck or handout materials, the room's location and layout, and the meeting agenda and invitation list. The most persuasive presentations often follow a discussion-and-dialogue format, in which the speaker knows the material so well that she does not need to refer to slides or notes to convey the message or to answer questions from the audience.

EFFECTIVE WRITTEN COMMUNICATION

Although verbal communication is the most direct and intimate way to deliver a message, the ability for humans to retain all the intricacies of a complex verbal message is finite and can be affected by personal biases and interpretations. Written communication therefore becomes more significant on a long-term basis because it provides a message that staff can keep and review repeatedly. Messages in writing thus provide great advantages, but they also carry inherent risks: Written communications lack the assistance of facial expressions, body language, and voice inflection, and they can easily be misinterpreted if not carefully planned and executed. The fact that written messages endure in perpetuity can also have human resource and legal implications if such messages are fired off in a haphazard manner. The following protocol, which is summarized in Exhibit 10.4, can help leaders communicate more effectively in writing.

The following framework can assist in crafting effective written messages:
1. Be selective in using written communication.
2. Develop a mental checklist.
3. Consider timing.
4. Use a clear and personal writing style.
5. Be generous with handwritten notes.

Be Selective in Using Written Communication

Written communications addressed to large groups are impersonal and should be reserved for such purposes as general information sharing (e.g., announcing an upcoming employee forum), implementing policy changes that need to be communicated widely and referenced in the future, and providing in-depth, complicated, or technical information. When written communications are used to thank others, the messages should be handwritten and individually addressed, and they should contain specific information on the reason for thanks. Personal communications that have the potential to become emotionally charged should generally be handled face to face.

Develop a Mental Checklist

Before writing, leaders should use a mental outline to map out why they are writing, the specific message they wish to convey, to whom they are writing, the appropriate writing style to underscore the desired message, and the appropriate writing format (e.g., formal memo, letter, informal note). In recent years, e-mail has become the quickest and most frequently used format for sending written messages; however, leaders should be aware that e-mail generally does not offer the same impact as personally handwritten notes and does not have the confidentiality of traditional written formats. Leaders should exercise caution in choosing the appropriate format when sending written communications.

Consider Timing

The timing of written communications is often more important than the content. Messages drafted when one is angry, upset, or tired can lead to embarrassing exchanges that the sender will soon regret. Remember this simple but critical point: Written communications—especially e-mails—last forever, and they can be easily shared or forwarded. In emotionally charged situations, a leader often benefits from allowing time to pass before committing a message to writing.

Use a Clear and Personal Writing Style

Consistency is one of the hallmarks of professionalism, and it is especially important in executive communication. The written "voice" in which executives express themselves reflects who they are as people and as leaders. Effective leaders know that their writing needs to be a genuine representation of their personality and leadership style. A leader who is affable and approachable but uses an aggressive and abrupt writing style will create cognitive dissonance with staff. As with verbal communication, leaders should be concise and clear in their written communications. They should avoid jargon, use concrete language, and be direct and to the point. Many executives make the mistake of using lengthy, complicated statements when simpler wording would be more effective—for instance, giving the direction to "terminate this employee" is less prone to misinterpretation than "give due consideration to ending the employment relationship with the aforementioned employee." Readers might enjoy this sentence that was actually used in a physician leadership-development workbook: "There are a large number of physicians, usually specialists and sub-specialists, who find significant challenges and difficulties with their abilities to maintain an appropriate sense of balance in their communications during interactions with others because typically and historically they have worked and practiced medicine in situations where most of what they say and communicate is involved with one-way messages and environments where feedback is rarely given." An effective communicator might make the point more clearly: "Many physicians are poor listeners."

Be Generous with Handwritten Notes

Handwritten notes clearly demonstrate that a busy executive has made an extra effort to send personal communication to the individual receiving the note. A note of thanks, sympathy, or congratulations sent from an executive to an employee's home can make a tremendous impression on the employee. It can create a loyalty that far outweighs the few moments needed for the leader to write the message.

TECHNOLOGY AND COMMUNICATION

Exciting advances in information technology have dramatically increased the speed and convenience of communication. Today, e-mail, Skype, and social media enable executives to break down geographic boundaries and communicate rapidly and broadly with employees. To remain competitive in a rapidly changing world, leaders must keep abreast of the latest trends in information technology and determine how to best use this technology. This chapter's opening vignette demonstrates how social media can provide powerful mechanisms for spreading messages and creating momentum—for good or bad—among employees. Leaders must make informed decisions about when to introduce technology to facilitate communication and how to set appropriate guidelines so that the technology does not endanger information security or cause productivity loss. The following protocols, which are summarized in Exhibit 10.5, can assist leaders in appropriately using technology to enhance communication in their organizations.

EXHIBIT 10.5: Protocol for Effective Use of Technology in Communication

The following framework can assist in effectively using technology to enhance communication:

1. Set guidelines for technology use during meetings.
2. Be responsive and timely.
3. Understand appropriate uses of social media.
4. Apply the *New York Times* test.

Set Guidelines for Technology Use During Meetings

With the proliferation of smartphone technology, the sight of people texting, responding to e-mail, or even surfing the web has become a ubiquitous distraction in all businesses, including healthcare. Quite simply, writing or reading e-mails or text messages during meetings or other work-related functions sends the wrong signals to others. Even if you think you are being discreet, others will notice you hunching over your cell phone when you are supposed to be paying attention. This behavior is rude, may cause you to miss important information, and curbs your ability to contribute in a meaningful way to the discussion. Unless you are administrator on call and need to respond to an immediate crisis, the messages can wait until the meeting is over. Many CEOs have adopted "no cell phone" meetings.

Be Responsive and Timely

Most leaders receive numerous messages on a daily basis through a variety of media, and many of these messages contain complex information, considerable data, and requests for action. Leaders should respond to all such messages in a timely manner. Leaders should not be so eager to clear out their inboxes that they respond definitively to messages without fully reviewing the information, but they must not let the messages languish. The most successful leaders develop methods to skim and triage their messages and try to respond to all e-mails within 24 hours.

Understand Appropriate Uses of Social Media

In the early days of Myspace and Facebook, healthcare organizations generally took a hard-line approach that banned all social media use by employees during work hours. Since that time, however, most organizations' social media policies have evolved. Used properly, social media can be a powerful tool to enhance communication, strengthen an organization's reputation, and develop a robust professional network. Nearly all hospitals now take a more proactive approach to social media. Most host Facebook and Twitter accounts, which allow leaders to share announcements of special events and exciting patient stories with the communities being served. Social media accounts also enable leaders to respond quickly to any negative comments posted online regarding the organization's services. Professional networks such as LinkedIn allow busy leaders to stay in touch and build new relationships in an industry in which leaders change employers frequently. Leaders should embrace the positive aspects of social media tools to advance their careers and professional reputations. However, some caution is in order: Personal social media use should occur only after normal working hours and outside of the office, and leaders should never share or post sensitive information about their employers or patients. Leaders at all times are visible representatives of the organizations they serve, so they should hold themselves to a high standard on their personal sites. Pictures on a Facebook page showing a leader in risqué clothing or drinking alcohol with friends can not only prove embarrassing to the organization; they can also limit the individual's employment options for the future.

Apply the *New York Times* Test

Before writing an e-mail, sending a text, leaving a voicemail, or posting a comment online, ask yourself this fundamental question: Would you mind seeing that message published on the front page of the *New York Times*? If your answer is yes, you should reconsider the message. The facts are clear: Numerous professional careers have been harmed by an embarrassing photo on Facebook, an e-mail sent in haste, a false statement on LinkedIn, or a problematic tweet on Twitter. Electronic communication is permanent, is discoverable in a court of law, and has great likelihood of being shared. *Do not* write anything that you would not want to see become public. Frankly, considering how frequently this precept is violated, we suggest that readers read it once again. Consider the suggestions in Exhibit 10.6. In addition, see Appendix B for more in-depth suggestions for maximizing the value of LinkedIn without violating appropriate behavior.

SUMMARY

Effective communication is perhaps the most critical and most challenging skill set that leaders in any industry must master. Leaders may be brilliant strategists with plans to catapult their organizations to national prominence, but failure to communicate these

EXHIBIT 10.6: Professional Guidance on the Use of Social Media

1. Think before you post.
2. Ask yourself this question: Do you really want profile information that is political, is publicly sensitive, or may reflect negatively on your job or career?
3. Pictures used on *any* site should be professional. Definitely use a professional picture on LinkedIn.
4. Guard your professionalism by monitoring what others post about you and "untag" photos that may be inappropriate.
5. Be cautious when accepting friend requests.
6. Do not join unprofessional groups.
7. Make sure your language is not considered obscene or offensive.
8. Use privacy settings to ensure confidentiality.
9. Finally, although many social media sites are "personal" in nature, the reality is that leaders give up certain rights along these lines. Be cautious about what you share and what is shared about you.

strategies in a clear and compelling manner can lead them to failure. *Leadership* can be defined as the process of influencing others toward common goals. The abilities to influence, inspire, persuade, and deliver effective messages are inextricably linked to all the core competencies that every healthcare leader must possess. Dye and Garman (2015, 50) write, "As important as vision is, it will not move an organization where it needs to go without systematic and compelling communication."

GUEST COMMENTARY: JEREMY C. ADAMS

Digital communication tools amplify any signal sent by a leader, whether good or bad. Leaders therefore must carefully consider the type and content of messages they send and remain attuned to digital media's risks

(continued)

(continued from previous page)

and pitfalls. A leader's lazy, one-word reply to an e-mail, for instance, might initiate hours of unnecessary effort by subordinates. A smartphone's "autocorrect" typing system might drastically alter the content of a brief Twitter post seen by thousands. Public trust can be eroded instantly when a leader communicates an opinion or political position over social media that is at odds with organizational values.

At the same time, digital media, when used in a positive manner, can expand career opportunities, increase employee engagement, and help retain customers. Intranet articles and blog posts allow leaders to distribute long-form content—materials that might be overlooked if sent via e-mail—to interested followers. Platforms such as Twitter and YouTube allow leaders to communicate with many people at once without the delays of formal chains of command. A leader can use a variety of digital media tools to gain personal feedback, gauge public perception on a tough issue, or allow employees to report problems directly.

When using any digital communication platform, remember that what you communicate matters. It matters to you, it matters to the receiver, and it matters to all those who were not an intended receiver but still received the message all the same. Digital communication technology is a force multiplier—use it wisely.

Jeremy C. Adams
Senior Strategy and Planning Consultant
Cardinal Health, Inc.
Dublin, Ohio

REFLECTIVE QUESTIONS

1. What are your organization's policies on social media use? How could they be enhanced to facilitate more effective communication to staff and patients?

2. Using the protocols presented in the chapter, develop your own "mental checklist" to guide your e-mails and other written communications. How can this tool be used to improve the quality of your written communications going forward?

3. Do you have social media posts, pictures, blogs, or messages that might be considered unprofessional?

RESOURCES AND EXERCISES FOR LEADERSHIP DEVELOPMENT

1. Many websites provide communications exercises to be used by trainers. Seek out these sites and try some of the exercises at an employee meeting. Use the exercises to generate discussion about the quality of communications within the work group.

2. Do you feel that gender differences drive different communication styles? Before concluding with an answer, consider the views of Simma Lieberman (www.simmalieberman.com/articles/maleandfemale.html) and the American Psychological Association (www.apa.org /research/action/difference.aspx).

3. Take one of the more common style tests, such as the Myers-Briggs Type Indicator, the Keirsey Bates test, or the Personalysis. (Some tests are available in abbreviated versions online: www.capt.org/take-mbti-assessment /mbti.htm; www.keirsey.com/sorter/register.aspx; www

.humanmetrics.com/cgi-win/jtypes2.asp.) Have your spouse or good friends take the same test and compare results. How do your communication styles compare?

4. Social media have become a pervasive part of life. Gather a group of peers and discuss the various ways in which social media can be helpful or harmful. To what extent does everyone agree?

5. Review the following books related to social media:

> Golden, M. 2010. *Social Media Strategies for Professionals and Their Firms: The Guide to Establishing Credibility and Accelerating Relationships.* Hoboken, NJ: Wiley.

> Lipschultz, J. H. 2014. *Social Media Communication: Concepts, Practices, Data, Law and Ethics.* New York: Routledge.

REFERENCES

Dye, C. F., and A. N. Garman. 2015. *Exceptional Leadership: 16 Critical Competencies for Healthcare Executives*, 2nd ed. Chicago: Health Administration Press.

Robles, M. M. 2012. "Executive Perceptions of the Top 10 Soft Skills Needed in Today's Workplace." *Business Communication Quarterly* 75 (4): 453–565.

CHAPTER 11

Physician Relationships

Nothing replaces the ability to get to know physicians on a personal and more intimate basis. This exercise of time will go a long way toward reducing misunderstandings and conflict situations.

—Jacque Sokolov, MD

Guide to Reader

Practically every healthcare leader will agree that success is often more directly correlated with strong physician relationships than with anything else. Candidly, your authors believe that, after those dealing with ethics and people relationships, the protocols in this chapter may be the most essential to a long, flourishing career in healthcare.

The Broken Partnership

In response to the changing landscape of a postreform environment, the leadership team of a successful pediatric hospital in a rapidly growing metropolitan area decided that the organization's strategic plan needed an overhaul. Historically, the organization had enjoyed success with a "Switzerland" approach: It provided its highly specialized services broadly, accepted referrals from all the providers in the area, and did not formally partner with any single system so as not to alienate potential referral streams.

Recently, however, the large, integrated systems in the area had begun developing delivery mechanisms that would facilitate population health management across the continuum of care, and accountable care organizations (ACOs) emerged. As this shift occurred, the pediatric facility was approached several times with offers to be the pediatric content experts and care provider for nearly every adult care system in the region. The hospital leadership decided that their historical position as "Switzerland," in which they did not formally partner with any system, needed to evolve to a new approach in which they would be willing to partner with any system that asked them to provide services. The rationale was that, if they served as the pediatric "plug-in" for ACOs in the area, the sponsoring systems would be less likely to develop competing pediatric services. With this strategy in mind, the leadership of the pediatric facility signed a series of strategic partnership documents with multiple systems to provide everything from telemedicine consults in rural areas to oversight of inpatient pediatric services.

The change in strategy was universally applauded by the leadership of the pediatric hospital. However, the

(continued)

(continued from previous page)

leaders had failed to include their academic partner in the discussion, and the faculty and residents in the Department of Pediatrics provided over 90 percent of the patient care delivered in the facility. The chairman of pediatrics not only was offended by not being included in the strategic discussions, but he also did not agree with the direction of the multiple affiliations and made his displeasure known to his medical staff colleagues.

The situation came to a head when the CEO of the pediatric facility agreed to develop a pediatric multispecialty clinic on the new campus of a large adult-based care facility. A facility was built, the center's administrator and staff were hired, and a grand opening was planned. One month prior to the opening, however, the chairman of pediatrics refused to provide any physician coverage to the center. Because the Department of Pediatrics had an exclusive agreement to provide all medical services for the facility, the CEO was left with a fully staffed clinic but no providers to see patients. This standoff continued for over a year, after which the hospital CEO gave up and sold the property. Nearly every partnership formed by the hospital leaders ultimately failed, all due to poor communication and relationship development with their physician partners.

Be mindful: There are few professions that have experienced greater fundamental changes in recent years than serving as a physician. With incentives now pushing physicians toward increased engagement with hospitals, healthcare leaders must actively engage physicians in strategy development, governance, and operations to ensure that these newly formed partnerships are successful.

CHANGING PHYSICIAN DYNAMICS

To the general public, physicians are the most visible and respected representation of healthcare. They serve as gatekeepers to healthcare access and are responsible—either directly or through mid-level providers—for every prescription, admission, and procedure. Because physicians drive billions of dollars in revenues and costs, a leader's ability to influence their behavior can be a powerful change agent in improving quality and efficiency in an organization and growing services to meet the needs of a community. Leaders who hope to gain support for their strategies must cultivate positive professional and interpersonal relationships with physicians; otherwise, they risk the same kind of disconnect highlighted in the vignette.

In the United States, the federal government has determined that the best way to fundamentally shift the healthcare delivery paradigm is through greater alignment and collaboration between healthcare leaders and their physician partners. As a result, healthcare reform laws have set forth incentives to encourage physician and hospital integration. For example, with measures that hold hospitals fiscally accountable for preventing readmissions—even though hospitals control only a small portion of the factors contributing to readmissions—the focus of hospital leadership broadens from providing acute care services to working upstream and downstream with physician partners to more effectively manage the continuum of care. In addition, innovative reimbursement models, such as accountable care organizations and bundled payment mechanisms, introduce dynamics in which hospitals and physicians share financial risk for delivering care to a population of patients. Today, the financial viability of physician practices and the ongoing success of healthcare delivery systems are inextricably linked.

This new era of collaboration follows a period in which systematic changes in healthcare moved the interests of hospitals and physicians in opposite directions. Many health systems employed physicians in the 1990s as a defense mechanism to managed care, and some divested them a few years later after suffering financial losses. Physicians in some areas of the country created large independent practice associations and group practices to leverage their strength with third-party payers. Many eschewed tighter integration with hospitals. With more procedures moving to the outpatient setting, a large number of physicians invested in ambulatory surgery centers and surgical hospitals. As the use of hospitalists grew (see Exhibit 11.1), primary care physicians became less involved in hospital operations as they gave up call coverage in favor of outpatient-only practices.

Changes in healthcare now present new motivations to rebuild hospital–physician relationships. Physicians faced with stagnant reimbursement rates, higher overhead, and dealings with third-party payers are seeking alignment with healthcare systems for greater work–life balance and increased security. Hospitals are shifting their focus from acute care to integrated delivery systems in an effort to maximize reimbursement structures based on quality,

EXHIBIT 11.1: Hospitals Using Hospitalists, by Region

Region	Percentage of Hospitals Reporting Use of Hospitalists
New England	84.9%
Mid-Atlantic	73.0%
South Atlantic	72.6%
East North Central	64.8%
East South Central	64.9%
West North Central	32.0%
West South Central	49.1%
Mountain	61.1%
Pacific	73.4%

Source: Data from American Hospital Association (2012).

outcomes, efficiency, and appropriate utilization patterns. These dynamics have led to a rapid increase in the formal alignment of physicians with hospitals and healthcare systems. This alignment can run the gamut from medical directorships to professional services agreements to clinical comanagement of service lines to participation in hospital-sponsored ACOs. More frequently, however, physicians and hospitals are moving to employment as the preferred method of integration. Since 2008, physicians in private practice have become a minority in the United States, and their percentage continues to shrink every year.

Closer relationships and employment arrangements, however, do not always produce desired alignment around cost control, quality, or growth; therefore, healthcare leaders must continue to focus their energies on building effective physician relationships. An effective working relationship requires mutual collaboration, an understanding of the value that both executives and physicians

---

EXHIBIT 11.2: Four Ways to Connect with Physicians

Clinician/caregiver
"May I long experience the joy of healing those who seek my help." (Modern version of the Hippocratic Oath, by Louis Lasagna, MD, longtime dean of Tufts School of Medicine)

Professional friend
A wise CEO once said, "Get the physicians to know you first as a person. If physicians know you only as the representation of your 'office,' you will have struggles as you try to relate to them."

Business partner
Physicians of all specialties have business interests, and many strong relationships develop from business activities.

Customer
In a manner, the hospital is a workshop for the physician, and the healthcare leader should aim to provide for the physician's needs.

---

bring to the equation, and finesse. Leaders should recognize that physicians are both internal customers of the hospital and business partners with vested financial interests. The protocols in this chapter aim to enhance the understanding of physician motivation, in hopes that leaders can translate this enhanced understanding into more effective collaborative relationships.

Readers hoping to develop strong physician relationships are encouraged to view physicians in four ways: as clinicians/caregivers, as customers, as business partners, and as professional friends. These four dimensions, summarized in Exhibit 11.2, provide the framework for this chapter.

PHYSICIANS AS CLINICIANS/CAREGIVERS

Most physicians chose their careers to provide care, to heal, and to prevent disease. The Latin phrase *primum non nocere*— meaning *first do no harm*—provides a principal guide for physician behavior. The white coat ceremony for many physicians is a solemn event that initiates them into the care of patients. Developing strong relationships with physicians requires an appreciation for their caregiver focus and an understanding of related rituals and customs.

However, even though the majority of physicians share a common purpose and customs, physicians are unique individuals and should be approached as such by healthcare leaders. Dye and Sokolov (2013, 13) summarize this point well: "Doctors are not a homogeneous group. In looking at how to achieve strategic management objectives, you have to be aware of the expectations for the different physician populations that are critical to the enterprise or organizational success as a whole. There is too often a tendency to say, 'This guy is a doctor, so he will be overfocused on clinical and be totally impractical.' But at the end of the day, that may be far from it. Those kinds of stereotypical characterizations will work against you in building effective leadership."

PHYSICIANS AS CUSTOMERS

Physicians face overwhelming pressure from the increased transparency of data around outcomes and customer satisfaction and from the higher level of consumerism driven by this new access to information. Patients often rely on physicians' recommendations for which hospital or health system to use, and physicians risk losing credibility if their patients have bad experiences. Healthcare leaders therefore must create an environment that actively engages physician partners, honors their time and commitment to safe patient care, and is efficient and customer friendly. Leaders should serve the physicians, look after their interests, and, essentially, connect with physicians as customers themselves. Physicians are constantly courted by competing healthcare organizations to redirect patient volume, and leaders must know what other organizations are offering and be as competitive as possible. Executives should provide physicians with clear, up-to-date, and concise information about their organizations. Remember that physician needs are not always related to new equipment or the latest "gadgets"; often they are focused on the patient experience and on the physician's ability to have a voice in shaping the hospital's future. The following protocol, summarized in Exhibit 11.3, can assist leaders in creating a physician-friendly environment.

EXHIBIT 11.3: Protocol for Physician Customer Service

The following framework can assist in creating a physician-friendly environment:

1. Honor the physician's role.
2. Develop and maintain healthy relationships.
3. Involve physicians in strategy.
4. Be flexible and responsive.
5. Manage well.

Honor the Physician's Role

Physicians are the ultimate content experts on clinical matters and are by nature very bright individuals. Nonetheless, they serve in a profession under great stress. The *Wall Street Journal* reported that only 6 percent of physicians in a national survey described their morale as positive and that 84 percent said their incomes were constant or decreasing (Jauhar 2014). Even more telling, a majority of doctors said they would discourage a friend or family member from entering the profession. A prevailing negative attitude has been driven by disillusionment with reimbursement, compensation, patient attitudes, and social stature. Such circumstances place even greater importance on the need for leaders to reinforce and bolster the role of physicians as both clinical experts and patient advocates. It is not enough to give them cookies on National Doctors' Day; physicians every day should be shown the respect they deserve as the caregivers of our patients. The following actions can assist in this regard:

- *Avoid making clinical decisions.* Executives who are not physicians should not address or intervene in clinical decisions; they instead should defer to, or at least consult with, their physician partners. An increasing number of organizations use chief medical officers who can serve as a formal liaison and "translator" between the executive team and physicians. The learning point here is simple and clear: Nonclinicians must not step into clinical matters.
- *Accept that physicians are patient advocates.* Most physicians take extremely seriously their oaths to care for patients, and they consider their bond with their patients to be a sacred one. The relationships that grow between physicians and patients often put the doctors in a patient advocacy role, which can translate into requests by physicians for

new programs, equipment, and services. Leaders should give all such requests due consideration. A number of organizations use physician review committees to guide the purchase of capital and patient-related equipment; such committees can help mitigate possible conflicts.

Develop and Maintain Healthy Relationships

Too often, invisible barriers develop within healthcare organizations between the people in executive offices and the physicians caring for patients. Leaders should recognize the risks in this dynamic and actively work to foster positive relationships with caregivers. These relationships must allow for open and honest dialogue about issues that are important to practicing physicians. Leaders should be visible in patient care areas and should periodically have lunch or breakfast in the physician lounge or dining room; doing so maintains a sense of approachability and involvement. Federal laws place strict limits on the amount of money executives can spend in interactions with doctors, but taking influential physicians and their spouses out to dinner occasionally is still acceptable. A leader can use such outings to build personal connections with physicians outside the confines of the business setting. Other suggestions for building healthy relationships include the following:

- *Establish a physician liaison position.* Even the smallest of hospitals should consider the establishment of a physician liaison position as an investment critical to ongoing success. The primary roles of the liaison are to befriend the physician office staff, to identify small issues that could grow into major sources of dissatisfaction, and to be aware of physician thoughts and plans. The liaison(s) must have access to key organizational decision makers and be highly visible to physician office staff members.

- *Survey physicians frequently.* Surveying physicians regularly—either through formal electronic processes (such as SurveyMonkey) or through focus group discussions—can help identify physician concerns and interests, improve physician satisfaction, and enhance relationships. Once concerns have been identified, executives should address those concerns as quickly as is practical and communicate resolutions back to the physicians in a timely manner.

Involve Physicians in Strategy

The healthcare systems that will maximize the opportunities set forth by the Affordable Care Act will be those that enjoy tight integration with their physician partners and a shared vision for the future. Dye and Sokolov (2013, 26) write, "The future healthcare enterprise is one in which physicians will be actively involved in setting strategic direction and managing day-to-day operations. Ultimately, all the incentives will be aligned because the physician enterprise and the business enterprise that manages health, wellness, and sickness will be one and the same." The most effective way to create this shared vision is to involve physician leaders in the development of strategy. Medical staff members are often confused or not fully informed about certain implications of healthcare reform, and in the absence of factual information, they often will draw their own conclusions about executives' motivations for strategic initiatives. Giving the physicians a meaningful place at the planning table is a sign of respect, and it reinforces the role of physicians as the clinical content experts for the organization.

Be Flexible and Responsive

Physicians are extremely busy and often manage several priorities at once. The same could be said of healthcare executives, but physicians also balance decisions and obligations that have dramatic impacts on patient outcomes. Many physicians feel that administrative meetings can interfere with their clinical duties and their responsibilities to patients. To minimize this sense of disruption, leaders should be respectful of physicians' busy schedules and competing priorities. The following actions, emphasizing flexibility and responsiveness, can help leaders demonstrate this respect:

- *Accommodate the physician's schedule.* Executives should realize that most physicians—even those employed by a health system—earn their income based on productivity. As a result, meetings and delays in schedules translate into lower personal paychecks. When scheduling meetings with doctors, ensure that the meetings are scheduled at times convenient for the physicians, that they start and end on time, and that they are effectively managed.

- *Respond quickly and follow up.* The requests and questions that leaders receive from physicians are not always easy, and they often lack straightforward answers. Nonetheless, executives should prioritize these communications and respond in a timely manner. Because physicians are generally fact-driven people, responses should be well thought out. Any decision, policy, or process change should have a clear rationale. Remember that physicians are trained to ask questions and to probe further into explanations; realize that they do so not out of disrespect but out of a genuine effort to understand issues that affect their practices.

Manage Well

At the end of the day, physicians respect action and results. They want a safe and high-quality environment for patients, a staff of highly skilled nurses and clinicians, an efficient place to practice, and access to current technologies and supplies. Leaders will ultimately be judged on how their organization is run and on what kind of environment they create. If executives deliver on promises and create a leadership team that effectively executes on the organization's strategies, enhanced trust between physicians and their administrative counterparts will result.

PHYSICIANS AS BUSINESS PARTNERS

Partnerships between healthcare organizations and physicians have developed at an accelerated pace and taken a variety of new forms, and this trend looks only to increase in the future postreform environment. Traditional forms of alignment, such as medical directorships and physician–hospital organizations (PHOs), have given way to new structures such as clinically integrated organizations (CIOs), accountable care organizations (ACOs), service line comanagement agreements, and employment models. Each of these structures has various legal requirements intended to allow physicians and hospitals to partner more closely, with the aims of improving quality and reducing costs. Many such partnerships have failed, and many failures have resulted from interpersonal conflict, a lack of shared vision, conflicts of interest, misaligned financial incentives, and poor organizational culture. The protocol that follows, which is summarized in Exhibit 11.4, describes a new leadership mind-set that can help ease tensions when dealing with physician business partners.

EXHIBIT 11.4: Protocol for Physician Business Partnerships

The following framework can assist in creating strong business relationships with physicians:

1. Be fair, just, and honest.
2. Create stability in leadership.
3. Balance risk and structural models.

Be Fair, Just, and Honest

Questions of fairness, and the perceptions surrounding fairness, can be problematic in any partnership. Such concerns are compounded if an inherent distrust already exists among the parties. Leaders should take great care to be open and honest in their business dealings. They should clearly spell out all parameters of business relationships in writing so that misunderstandings can be managed and legal risks minimized. Procedural justice methods should be in place so that individuals can formally question or challenge actions that affect them without fear of retaliation.

Create Stability in Leadership

Many physicians perceive executives as frequent job changers. In the words of one physician to a new CEO, "I've seen a lot of you come and a lot of you go, and I figure I will outlast you just like I have the others." Although more recent generations have shown increasing mobility, most physicians remain in a single location for their entire professional careers. As a result, they often have a healthy dose of skepticism when they hear an executive say she is committed to the long-term success of a new partnership structure.

With any alignment structure, executives must be transparent with physicians. To the extent possible, leaders should share growth goals, strategic initiatives, and competitive matters openly with their physician partners. Moreover, boards should involve physicians in formal succession-planning processes for organizational leadership, especially if various partnerships are in place with physicians. Giving physicians a say in leadership changes in partnership organizations brings a sense of stability and helps to alleviate doctors' concerns during transitions.

Balance Risk and Structural Models

Executives represent healthcare organizations that have imposing resources and access to significant capital. However, because executives have a limited personal stake in the organizations' business dealings, their risks are relatively low. Physicians know this. Executives encounter partnership transactions frequently, but physicians do not. And more important, physicians enter into contracts and agreements as individuals, and they often pledge personal assets to back the transactions. The success or failure of a venture often depends on a physician's personal skills or training, and failure can result in personal financial loss for the physician. Leaders should keep these circumstances in mind and offer an alignment model that minimizes risk exposure for physicians while still accomplishing the goals of the organization.

PHYSICIANS AS PROFESSIONAL FRIENDS

To put it bluntly, many nonclinical administrators are afraid of physicians. They perceive that physicians have a certain "mystique" and hold a more substantive position in the healthcare world. To be sure, this perception to some extent is fed by physicians, many of whom are dissatisfied with their administration and wish to gain the upper hand with leaders and managers. When rivalries escalate, executives sometimes react with name calling and negative characterizations: For instance, they might compare the task of leading physicians to "herding cats," claim that "physician leadership is an oxymoron," or portray doctors as money hungry. One unnamed CEO was heard complaining that physicians "are selfish, self-centered, arrogant, poor listeners, and downright disruptive."

Quotes attributed to one particularly derogatory article about physicians, titled "How to Discourage a Doctor," have circulated online, and readers are urged to take note of its deeply flawed advice for executives (Gunderman 2014): "Merely controlling the purse strings is not enough. To truly seize the reins of medicine, it is necessary to do more, to get into the heads and hearts of physicians. And the way to do this is to show physicians that they are not nearly so important as they think they are. Physicians have long seen the patient–physician relationship as the very center of the healthcare solar system. As we go forward, they must be made to feel that this relationship is not the sun around which everything else orbits, but rather one of the dimmer peripheral planets, a Neptune or perhaps Uranus." The article offers suggestions to executives: "Make healthcare incomprehensible to physicians. . . . Promote a sense of insecurity among the medical staff. A comfortable physician is a confident physician, and a confident physician usually proves difficult to control. To undermine confidence, let it be known that physicians' jobs are in jeopardy and their compensation is likely to decline." The approach described in this article is surely *not* the recipe for positive physician relationships. The fact that the piece appeared in 2014 and continues to be posted in medical staff lounges is cause for concern.

Leaders who have developed strong physician relationships— and those who have mastered the protocols in this chapter—describe physicians very differently. Effective leaders view physicians first as individuals with whom they expect to develop professional friendships. The concepts listed throughout this chapter are all important, but this foundational precept is the most crucial. Will every physician become a professional friend? No. But successful leaders will count many physicians in that category.

The guidelines for professional friendships with physicians are simple, and they are presented in Exhibit 11.5. First, leaders should seek to understand, as Covey (2013) taught in his famous work, *The 7 Habits of Highly Successful People*. Effective leaders need a deep understanding of physicians' educational processes, their scientific tendencies, and the ways they think and process information. Next, leaders must demonstrate professional respect. Comments like the "herding cats" remark mentioned previously are completely inappropriate. Leaders also must honor physicians' role in patient care and their commitment to the curing profession. Next, leaders should frequently visit physicians in the medical staff lounge, in patient care areas, and in physicians' private offices. A final suggestion is to support physicians, both professionally and personally. This support can involve a financial donation to a physician's community activity or philanthropic effort, or simply a donation of time to the physician's efforts. Note the absence of social and athletic activities in this list. These activities, though important, cannot be the sole efforts providing the basis for friendships; if they are, physicians may sense a lack of authenticity.

EXHIBIT 11.5: Developing Professional Friendships with Physicians
1. Learn about physicians.
2. Show them professional respect.
3. Revere their place at the center of patient care.
4. Visit them in their workshop.
5. Support them.

SUMMARY

The incentives and structures set forth through healthcare reform provide exciting opportunities for physicians and healthcare organizations to partner more closely, to collaborate around quality and efficiency, and to share in the financial rewards for improved performance. Collaborative relationships provide the key to more effective coordination of care and to meaningful reductions in the unnecessary utilization of resources. Leaders must remember that healthcare—regardless of any overarching corporate structure that may be in place—ultimately relies on building and maintaining trust and effective relationships with physician partners.

GUEST COMMENTARY: KENNETH H. COHN

When I teach my "Practical Strategies for Engaging Physicians" seminar for the American College of Healthcare Executives, participants can be differentiated by their answer to the question, "What percentage of your time do you devote to hospital–physician relations?" Early healthcare careerists generally say 10–25 percent, whereas experienced hospital CEOs tell me 90–100 percent.

The vignette about the pediatric hospital leaders who failed to involve the department chair in strategic discussions brings to mind a comment by a physician from upstate New York: "When we are not at the table, we feel like we are on the menu." Relations with physicians can become something of a self-fulfilling prophecy: When one treats physicians as adults, one gets adult behavior in return. My reaction to the events in the vignette would not be directed as much to the CEO specifically as to the other members of the C-suite and the board, whom I would encourage to speak up. After all, the welfare of their community is at stake.

I believe that hospital administrators, nurses, allied healthcare professionals, and physicians all chose healthcare careers to make a difference in patients' lives. Like conjoined twins, the viability of hospitals and physician practices are inextricably linked. We agree on the *why*, which should help us bridge our differences on the *how*—assuming we use active, empathetic listening to depersonalize those differences. The best way to resolve complex issues is through face-to-face communication.

I also believe that our job descriptions are blurring, especially in light of the need to decrease readmissions and

(continued)

(continued from previous page)

hospital-acquired conditions. Therefore, I take issue with the statement that nonclinicians must not step into clinical matters. Instead, I would encourage hospital leaders to form physician advisory groups consisting of well-respected clinical champions and to use clinical events and related discussions to educate both the clinical and nonclinical sides on the individual patient care issues encountered by physicians and the organizational issues familiar to administrators. Hospital leaders who fear physicians might reframe physicians' anger as pain and ask in an empathetic fashion: "It sounds like the issue you just described is causing you a lot of pain. How can we work together to improve the practice environment for you?" Pulling a splinter out of a lion's paw is frightening, but such action can create a lifelong relationship based on trust and mutual respect.

Kenneth H. Cohn, MD
CEO, Healthcare Collaboration
Amesbury, Massachusetts

Note from the authors: Ken Cohn passed away on June 24, 2015. Ken was well known and respected by many in healthcare and contributed greatly to the American College of Healthcare Executives and Health Administration Press. We count him as a friend who left us far too soon.

REFLECTIVE QUESTIONS

1. Review the vignette at the beginning of this chapter. How could the leaders of the pediatric facility have worked more effectively with their physician partners to produce a better outcome?

2. Why might an executive opt for a service line comanagement model rather than an employment structure for alignment with a large specialist physician group?

3. How well do you know physicians? Their educational pathway? Their training and job pressures?

RESOURCES AND EXERCISES FOR LEADERSHIP DEVELOPMENT

1. "Walk a day in their shoes." If you are a nonclinical person, seek out a physician whom you can spend a full day shadowing.

2. Ensure that you have a firm understanding of the medical school educational process. Consider shadowing a medical student or resident during patient rounds.

3. Grand rounds and other educational events provide excellent opportunities to gain a deeper understanding of clinical issues and challenges. Attend these when possible.

4. One of the most popular physician authors of recent years has been—and continues to be—Atul Gawande, MD. His books are must-reads, and his presentations at health leadership conferences are always worthwhile. Attend a presentation if possible, and review his website (http://atulgawande.com/).

REFERENCES

American Hospital Association (AHA). 2012. *AHA Hospital Statistics, 2012 Edition*. Washington, DC: American Hospital Association.

Covey, S. R. 2013. *The 7 Habits of Highly Effective People: Powerful Lessons in Personal Change*, 25th anniversary ed. New York: Simon and Schuster.

Dye, C. F., and J. J. Sokolov. 2013. *Developing Physician Leaders for Successful Clinical Integration*. Chicago: Health Administration Press.

Gunderman, R. 2014. "How to Discourage a Doctor." The Health Care Blog. Published September 18. http://thehealthcareblog.com/blog/2014/09/18/how-to-discourage-a-doctor/.

Jauhar, S. 2014. "Why Doctors Are Sick of Their Profession." *Wall Street Journal*. Published August 29. www.wsj.com/articles/the-u-s-s-ailing-medical-system-a-doctors-perspective-1409325361.

CHAPTER 12

Recruitment and Selection

No matter how good or successful you are, or how clever or crafty, your business and its future are in the hands of the people you hire.

—Akito Morita

Guide to Reader

The ability to attract, assess, and select the right team members is essential for any leader. These functions are commonly considered the responsibility of the human resources department, but every leader needs to learn the nuances of recruitment.

A Poorly Managed Process

A talented hospital vice president began interviewing at a competing hospital much larger than her own, seeking a leadership position for which she felt well qualified. The role was similar in scope to her current job, but the size of the organization compelled her to consider the lateral move. Her initial interview with the hospital COO took place in January, and it went well. She was told on the spot that she was one of the strongest candidates for the position and that she would definitely be included in the next round of interviews.

In February, the candidate had not heard back, so she called the COO to check on the status of the search. The COO apologized for the lack of progress and expressed his continued interest in her as a candidate. A few days later, she was scheduled for another round of interviews with various executives at the hospital. Because she was a local candidate, the interviews were sprinkled over a span of 15 days rather than conveniently scheduled together. The candidate complied and came in for all the interviews, but because she was taking so much time away from her current job and meeting with so many local executives, the confidentiality of her candidacy had been compromised. In addition, the candidate was left to find her own way to the executives' offices, most of the interviews began late, and several were poorly coordinated. One appointment began 40 minutes after the appointed time, making the candidate late for a meeting at her current hospital.

In April, the COO informed the candidate that she was one of two finalists and that she would next be interviewed by

(continued)

(continued from previous page)

the hospital's industrial psychologist to determine her "fit" with the executive team. However, because the psychologist was out of town, the meeting could not be scheduled until three weeks later. The candidate doubted the relevance of the psychologist's interview and the tests she was to be given, but she complied with the requirement.

Nearly a month after the psychological testing, the COO informed the candidate that the hospital had selected the other finalist. The rejected candidate later learned that the hospital had hired an individual who lacked healthcare experience and was obviously less qualified for the role than she was. She felt that her disjointed interview experience and rushed sessions with the company's executives were contributing factors in the hospital's decision. Moreover, she highly resented the leadership team's haphazard treatment, which exposed her candidacy within her own organization.

Be mindful: The most lasting impression an executive leaves on an organization is in the staff and the leaders he recruits. Poor recruitment and selection practices convey disrespect toward candidates, lead to costly hiring mistakes, and reflect badly on the organization.

THE REVOLVING DOOR OF LEADERSHIP

Change in leadership within an organization is, by definition, a disruptive event. When new leaders are introduced, they often delay or alter key strategic initiatives as they become acclimated to their new roles. Moreover, because the culture of an organization is largely predicated on the styles and priorities of its leaders, turnover often brings fundamental shifts in the fabric of the workplace. Turnover can also be extremely costly. The Center for American Progress finds that the cost of losing and replacing an executive is up to 213 percent of the salary of the position (Boushey and Glynn 2012), and Cascio (2006) reports that the cost of replacing a worker is typically 1.5 to 2.5 times the worker's salary. Such cost estimates include money spent on recruitment, selection, and training as well as expenses related to lower productivity, poor employee morale, and potential loss of customers.

Studies of turnover vary in their estimates of the average tenure for a CEO at a hospital. Most agree it is less than 5 years, but some say it is less than 3.5 (Brown 2013). Overall hospital CEO turnover reached an all-time high of 20 percent in 2013, and it remained high at 18 percent the following year (American College of Healthcare Executives 2014, 2015). Compounding the problem is the fact that, whenever a CEO turns over, significant turnover is likely elsewhere in the senior leadership ranks.

The accelerated rate of turnover in healthcare has a variety of underlying causes (e.g., promotional opportunities, industry changes, retirement), but it can be partially attributed to the field's historically poor performance in recruitment, selection, and succession planning. The *Harvard Business Review* suggests that nearly 80 percent of all turnover is the result of poor hiring decisions (Stone 2015). Too often, healthcare organizations lack a systematic approach to hiring, rely too much on "chemistry," and use faulty methods of assessment (see Exhibit 12.1). Psychologist Robert Hogan (personal communication) has said that many employers have such invalid selection processes that they would be better off flipping a coin to decide whom to hire. In addition, studies have found that, at best, only a third of healthcare organizations have succession plans (Garman and Tyler 2007).

Most hiring processes rely on individual and group interviews as the basis for selection. However, the reliability of interviews as predictors of future job performance is limited. One Michigan State University study found that the typical interview panel

EXHIBIT 12.1: Common Causes of Poor Selection

1. No systematic approach to the selection process
2. Haphazard and flawed assessment methods
3. Allowing chemistry to carry too much weight in the hiring decision
4. Lack of clarity about the role of the job
5. Lack of clear performance metrics

increased the likelihood of selecting the best candidate by less than 2 percent (Hunter and Hunter 1984). The chief reason for this poor predictive ability is that humans are heavily biased creatures whose perceptions of candidates are influenced by preconceived notions. With the subjective nature of typical interview questions, even the most experienced and well-intentioned hiring managers have a subconscious tendency to favor people similar to themselves. This tendency may lead to relatively compatible, homogeneous teams, but it does little to ensure that the most qualified or talented individuals are selected for the jobs.

Healthcare executives will likely hold leadership roles in multiple organizations during the course of their careers, and their success will largely be determined by the quality of their recruitment and selection decisions. The protocols in this chapter are intended to assist leaders in developing structured methodologies to match the best candidates to key roles. They also aim to help leaders become strong candidates themselves.

EFFECTIVE CANDIDATE SELECTION

There is no greater legacy that a leader leaves her organization than the quality of the individuals she hires. Moreover, the more senior the position a leader holds, the more dependent she is on subordinates for the success of the strategic initiatives she champions. As we have discussed, however, internal biases can cause leaders to unwittingly overlook the most qualified candidates, and one poor selection decision can derail an organization and severely damage the hiring manager's credibility. The following protocol, summarized in Exhibit 12.2, aims to reduce the subjectivity of the selection process and increase the likelihood that chosen candidates will ultimately be successful.

EXHIBIT 12.2: Protocol for Candidate Selection

The following framework can provide guidance when selecting a candidate for a key role:

1. Understand the job.
2. Use a standardized hiring process.
3. Treat applicants as customers.
4. Honor confidentiality.
5. Strategically use executive search firms.
6. Frame the assessment of candidates against a model.

Understand the Job

Often, executives make flawed hiring decisions because they have not taken the time to truly understand the specific functions and key success factors of the roles for which they are hiring. Many such mistakes can be avoided if the organization performs a formal job analysis of every leadership role. A job analysis involves breaking a job down into logical parts; analyzing each job function according to the knowledge, skills, and attributes required for effective performance; and evaluating the behavioral attributes of individuals who have been successful in key roles. With job analyses, the hiring process becomes faster and more effective because job candidates are evaluated on a more objective and consistent set of criteria. The process also allows the hiring manager to provide candidates with a "realistic job preview." A preview that offers a thorough description of responsibilities can limit the number of "surprises" experienced by new hires when they take on their roles and can ultimately increase job satisfaction. Phillips (1998, 673) states that realistic job previews "were related to higher performance and to lower attrition from the recruitment process, initial expectations, voluntary turnover, and all turnover."

Use a Standardized Hiring Process

The candidate featured in this chapter's opening vignette was the victim of an organization that lacked a standard approach to the screening of candidates. Without a framework to guide hiring activities, busy executives tend to squeeze in recruitment activities around other competing priorities, making for a rushed and disjointed experience for interviewees. Organizations should develop standardized interview formats and candidate feedback tools that provide appropriate time for each candidate and truly assess the skills and competencies required for the open positions. Some organizations assign oversight of all interview-related activities to an executive sponsor—usually the chief human resources officer, though some organizations rotate the duty. Highly effective organizations also have a time-frame expectation for the vetting of candidates to ensure that the process moves swiftly. This level of rigor increases the objectivity of the process and creates a more favorable experience for candidates.

Treat Applicants as Customers

Healthcare is a small community, and stories of candidates' negative experiences with an organization can spread quickly and limit the organization's access to top talent in the future. Thus, leaders should show common courtesy and aim to enhance each candidate's "customer" experience. Every interview is an opportunity to build the reputation of your organization and your own reputation as a leader. When you conduct an interview, market your organization and its benefits so that the applicant leaves with a positive view, even if he ultimately is not selected for the job. The following are a few simple ways to set your organization apart:

- If a candidate is flying in from out of town, personally pick her up at the airport. If a personal pickup is not possible, arrange for proper transportation and call to make sure she has arrived safely.
- Speak with the manager of the hotel where the candidate is staying. Let the manager know the candidate is a "VIP" guest, and ask that the hotel staff pay close attention to the candidate's needs.
- Consider leaving a personal welcome card along with a small gift, such as a fruit basket, in the candidate's hotel room.
- Pay close attention to the needs of the candidate's spouse and family. Provide appropriate information about real estate markets and school systems prior to the visit, and put the family in touch with a company-sponsored real estate agent to answer any questions that may arise.

Honor Confidentiality

Although some candidates are relatively open with their present employers when considering other opportunities, most are not. Many fear retaliation or loss of employment if word gets out about them considering other positions. Recruiters therefore must make every effort to protect confidentiality at all costs. Even though hiring managers intuitively understand the importance of confidentiality, breaches occur frequently, especially in a small industry such as healthcare. Some executives are flippant about the issue and make casual reference calls without the candidate's knowledge; they may even rationalize their actions by assuming that applicants understood the risks they were taking when they began the process.

The risk of breaches of confidentiality increases when community members (such as trustees) and physicians are involved in the hiring process, because they may be less aware of the detrimental effects of informal inquiries. Once the formal checking of references begins, interviewers must make sure candidates understand the referencing process. At times, an interviewer may need to contact, with an applicant's permission, individuals other than those on the formal reference list. When such contacts occur, the hiring organization must underscore the importance of confidentiality.

Strategically Use Executive Search Firms

Hiring organizations can engage executive search firms in *retained search*, *contingency search*, or *fee-for-service* arrangements. In a retained search process, a search firm performs the recruiting functions for a leadership role—including the sourcing, screening, and presenting of qualified candidates—and works with the hiring manager and human resources function of the sponsoring organization to schedule candidate interviews and arrange travel. In return, the employer pays the firm a set fee and reimburses additional expenses incurred during the recruitment process. Payment is due regardless of whether the employer finds a suitable candidate through the firm or through its own means. Under a contingency search arrangement, an employer can engage several firms to source candidates, and a fee is paid to a firm only if a candidate identified by that firm is hired. In a fee-for-service arrangement, an employer contracts with a search firm to handle only parts of the recruiting process, such as screening candidates or checking references. The firm bills only for the services it has provided, whether or not a suitable candidate has been found.

Typically, retained search firms are more effective advocates for the hiring employer, whereas contingency search firms focus more on simply referring candidates for hire. Contingency firms do not provide the extensive screening that retained firms do, and they may not fully vet candidates. To ensure a successful search, employers should consider how a search firm might enhance their recruitment process and what type of firm and what type of contractual arrangement make the most sense. The guidelines provided in Exhibit 12.3 can assist in navigating through this complex process.

Frame the Assessment of Candidates Against a Model

Perhaps most important, leaders should use a formalized model to frame the assessment of candidates. Exhibit 12.4 shows a selection assessment model from Dye and Sokolov (2013) that, when used effectively, helps determine the factors to be used in hiring or promotion decisions. These factors become the "selection criteria" and should be considered with the appropriate weight given to each factor. Determining the criteria in advance helps minimize the bias problem that occurs when hiring managers allow personal chemistry to carry too much weight in the selection decision. Ultimately, the goal is to have a decision-making process that is well thought-out and minimizes subjectivity to the extent possible.

BECOMING A SUCCESSFUL CANDIDATE

Thomas Edison said that "good fortune often happens when opportunity meets with preparation," and this statement clearly applies to leaders who effectively manage their careers and set themselves apart from other candidates. Executives in the field should always be prepared for calls from other organizations and from search consultants, and they should take these calls even if they are not currently interested in another job. If leaders are not interested in the opportunity presented, they should try to provide two or three appropriate referrals to the caller. In all instances, leaders should treat these calls as opportunities to promote themselves and their

EXHIBIT 12.3: Reasons for Using an Executive Search Firm

- Many employers do not have the time or expertise to appropriately source executive searches without outside help.
- A search firm often identifies candidates from a wider geographic area and a greater variety of organizations than the employer would on its own.
- Many potential candidates are not actively seeking employment, and the only way of reaching this candidate pool is through networks developed by search firms.
- A search firm can bring objectivity to the recruiting process, which can be helpful in vetting internal candidates.
- A search firm can help identify market salary ranges and peculiar aspects of a search that may not be immediately apparent to the employer.
- In some cases, an organization may need to begin a search confidentially to identify a candidate prior to the departure of the incumbent executive.
- A search firm consultant can provide additional management consulting, such as insights on organizational needs, what similar organizations are doing, and what leadership competencies can best address pressing system needs.

EXHIBIT 12.4: Selection Assessment Model

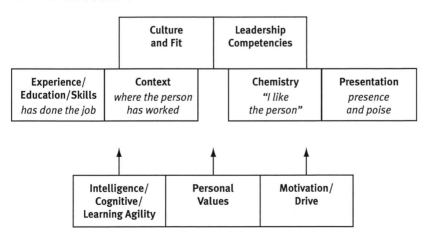

Source: Reprinted with permission from Dye and Sokolov (2013).

skill sets and to build relationships with search consultants and hiring managers. Such relationships enhance a leader's networking reach and help ensure calls in the future, when the timing may be right for a job move. Leaders looking to become successful candidates should consider the following protocol, which is summarized in Exhibit 12.5.

EXHIBIT 12.5: Protocol for Candidates

The following framework can provide guidance for candidates being considered for a key role:

1. Be informed.
2. Make a strong impression.
3. Professionally display your interest.
4. Be prepared for the expected questions.

Be Informed

The best way for a candidate to show that she takes the selection process seriously is to demonstrate a thorough knowledge of the hiring organization and the available role. Such knowledge not only conveys respect to the hiring executives; it also helps the candidate create advantages over other applicants and assess whether the role is a good fit personally and professionally. Most organizations and search firms provide extensive job specifications that describe the available position, its key goals, and the characteristics sought in the ideal candidate. Candidates should carefully review these documents and match their own experiences and talents with those desired for the role. Through this type of critical assessment, the candidate can develop specific talking points that are built around personal successes and relate to critical factors desired for the role. Candidates should learn as much as they can about the organization through publicly available data, and they should seek to understand the community the organization serves. Finally, when candidates receive details about the interview panel, they should run an Internet search of each interviewer to gain relevant background information and insight for preparation.

Make a Strong Impression

First impressions are never more important than during an interview. Candidates should arrive on time (actually a few minutes early), dress appropriately, bring hard copies of an updated resume and an organizational chart showing their current position, and be prepared to provide specific examples of applicable experiences. Candidates should greet all interviewers with a firm handshake, and they should maintain eye contact throughout each discussion. A proper balance between listening and speaking should allow candidates to "sell" themselves appropriately while still learning about the role. Candidates should also have a list of key questions to ask at the end of the interview to gain additional information; they can then compare the data with what has been provided by the search consultant.

Professionally Display Your Interest

Hiring executives tend to be extremely busy individuals, and recruitment processes, even for key leadership positions, sometimes must be placed on the back burner as pressing day-to-day issues arise. In follow-up communications to the hiring organization, candidates must strike a delicate balance. Those who communicate too little can appear apathetic, whereas those who communicate too much may be perceived as desperate. A good practice for after an interview is to personally send each interviewer a handwritten thank-you note. (An e-mail is appropriate as well but does not quite carry the same weight.) The note should convey your appreciation for the interviewer's time and succinctly recount your strengths and the reasons you would be a good fit for the team. Close the note by expressing your sincere interest in the position and your confidence in your ability to do the job well. Avoid making phone calls to the hiring organization. If you are working through a search firm, let the search consultant know of your ongoing interest, follow up regularly, and let the consultant be your conduit of communication with the hiring manager. A word of advice is in order regarding LinkedIn: Though it may be tempting to link with each person you met while interviewing, you should wait until a later time to do this, to avoid creating the wrong impression.

Be Prepared for the Expected Questions

Traditional interview staples such as "Tell me about yourself" and "What are your strengths and weaknesses?" still surface at times, but interviewers today have generally become more sophisticated. The most prevalent current approach is the *behavioral interview*, in which candidates are asked how they have actually handled or reacted to situations that are similar to situations likely to be faced in the job for which they are interviewing. Thus, candidates must be prepared to give specific examples of how they have handled various work events in the past. Additionally, the best behavioral interviews are also built around the key competencies that are essential to success on the job.

SUMMARY

The fundamental changes occurring in healthcare present leaders with new opportunities to make lasting impressions. Most of these opportunities will come with hiring decisions. Every healthcare organization in the United States is in the process of revamping its strategic plans, and each organization's ability to execute those plans will depend on the quality of organizational talent. The implications of recruiting and selecting the right candidates are vast. The most successful leaders will develop standardized processes to minimize personal biases and identify the most qualified individuals. At the same time, they will continuously prepare themselves for their own opportunities to contribute at a higher level.

REFLECTIVE QUESTIONS

1. Review the vignette at the beginning of the chapter. How could the hiring organization have improved its process to ensure that the candidate had a more positive experience?

2. Recall your last job interview. Regardless of whether you were selected, how could you have better prepared for the process and been a more effective candidate?

3. Call to mind a hiring mistake you have made. (If you have not made one yet, find a colleague who has and is willing to share.) Develop a list of actions that might have helped you avoid the error.

RESOURCES AND EXERCISES FOR LEADERSHIP DEVELOPMENT

1. Learn and master the practice of behavioral interviewing (i.e., asking questions that require the interviewee to describe specific past experiences as part of the answer). Doing so will help you both as an interviewer and as an interviewee. Behavioral interviewing is based on the principle that the best predictor of future behavior is a review of past behavior. For example, instead of asking, "How would you handle an angry physician?" an interviewer

would say, "Tell me about a specific time when you handled an angry physician, and give me some detail about how you managed the situation." The following online resources are worth reviewing:

- "Behavioral Interviewing: 'Back to the Future'" (2013) by M. A. Broscio (http://ache.org/pdf/secure/gifts/JA13 _careers_reprint.pdf)

- "Behavioral Interviewing" (2013) by the Virginia Tech Division of Student Affairs (www.career.vt.edu /interviewing/behavioral.html)

2. Review the following works concerning bias in selection:

- "Interviewer Biases" (2014) from the University of North Carolina School of the Arts (www.uncsa.edu /humanresources/forms/InterviewerBiases.pdf)

- "Cognitive Biases in Selection Decisions" (2011) by Cheng Wen Hua (www.cscollege.gov.sg/Knowledge /Pages/Cognitive-Biases-in-Selection-Decisions.aspx)

3. As noted earlier in the chapter, poor recruitment practices can be a barrier to successful hiring. Because recruitment is a process, the principles of Six Sigma and Lean may be used to help improve it. Begin with a review of the following website and then search for other Internet sources with suggestions for improvement: www.isixsigma .com/methodology/total-quality-management-tqm /case-study-improving-recruitment-processes-part-1-of-2/.

4. Disney is well known for its excellent hiring program. The Disney Institute (www.disneyinstitute.com) offers workshops on Disney's programs, and the institute's blog provides insight into some of Disney's principles (www .disneyinstitute.com/blog/2015/03/culture-101-why-its -important-to-hire-for-behaviors-as-well-as-skills/339/).

REFERENCES

American College of Healthcare Executives. 2015. "Hospital CEO Turnover Rate Remains Elevated." Published March 5. www.ache.org/pubs/Releases/2015/hospital-ceo-turnover-rate15.cfm.

————. 2014. "Hospital CEO Turnover Rate Increases." Published March 10. www.ache.org/pubs/Releases/2014/hospital_ceo_turnover_rate14.cfm.

Boushey, H., and S. J. Glynn. 2012. "There Are Significant Business Costs to Replacing Employees." Center for American Progress. Published November 16. www.americanprogress.org/issues/labor/report/2012/11/16/44464/there-are-significant-business-costs-to-replacing-employees/.

Brown, D. 2013. "Headhunters Charged to Replace Hospital CEOs with Innovative Industry Outsiders, Reveals Black Book Board Survey." Black Book Market Research. Published December 18. www.blackbookmarketresearch.com/headhunters-charged-to-replace-hospital-ceos-with-innovative-industry-outsiders-reveals-black-book-board-survey/.

Cascio, W. F. 2006. "The High Cost of Low Wages." *Harvard Business Review.* Published December. https://hbr.org/2006/12/the-high-cost-of-low-wages.

Dye, C. F., and J. J. Sokolov. 2013. *Developing Physician Leaders for Successful Clinical Integration.* Chicago: Health Administration Press.

Garman, A. N., and J. L. Tyler. 2007. "Succession Planning Practices & Outcomes in U.S. Hospital Systems: Final Report." American College of Healthcare Executives. Published August 20. www.ache.org/pubs/research/succession_planning.pdf.

Hunter, J. E., and R. F. Hunter. 1984. "Validity and Utility of Alternative Predictors of Job Performance." *Psychological Bulletin* 96 (1): 72–98.

Phillips, J. M. 1998. "Effects of Realistic Job Previews on Multiple Organizational Outcomes: A Meta-Analysis." *Academy of Management Journal* 41 (6): 673–90.

Stone, Z. 2015. "Taking the Pain Out of Employee Turnover." *USA Today.* Published May 26. www.usatoday.com/story/money /business/2015/05/26/ozy-employee-turnover/27956697/.

PART III

Serving Inside the Organization

CHAPTER 13

The New Position

Joining a new company is akin to an organ transplant—and you're the new organ. If you're not thoughtful in adapting to the new situation, you could end up being attacked by the organizational immune system and rejected.

—Michael C. Watkins

Guide to Reader

Since the publication of Watkins's (2003) *The First 90 Days: Critical Success Strategies for New Leaders at All Levels*, considerable attention has been placed on the ways that leaders take charge and establish themselves when they start in new positions. So much hinges on how individuals are introduced to the organization, how they learn the ropes, and how they begin to blend into the organizational culture. Move too quickly, and you may derail; move too slowly, and you may be ignored; move too aggressively, and you may be undermined. Identifying the unwritten expectations upon your arrival and managing them effectively are critical to your personal onboarding.

Seek First to Understand

An up-and-coming COO in a large not-for-profit hospital system was excited to be tapped for a president opening in one of the smaller facilities in the network. The facility had been acquired by the health system only a few months earlier, and the system CEO thought it would be the perfect proving ground for this talented young executive. The hospital was located in a small, rural community several miles from the system's flagship facility, and it had fallen on hard times recently because one of the town's major employers, a manufacturing plant for automotive parts, had shut down. The community was excited by the news of the acquisition, because many residents had feared the facility would close without assistance.

Eager to make a good impression, the newly minted president quickly implemented processes and procedures intended to bring the operations of the facility in line with those of the other facilities in the system. Convinced that the hospital's failure as a stand-alone facility was due to inept leadership, he systematically replaced several key executives. Within 90 days, 60 percent of the hospital's leadership positions were vacant. Talented new leaders were recruited, but these individuals had no history in the organization and were perceived as "outsiders" who had cost the staff's former colleagues their jobs. With such a massive exodus of leaders (some of whom had 20 years of tenure with the organization), high-performing staff members began questioning their job security and seeking employment elsewhere.

(continued)

(continued from previous page)

The new leadership team also began to implement significant changes in the operating model of the facility. Aware that the healthcare system had acquired the facility primarily to serve as a "feeder" hospital to the flagship facility, the team started winding down higher-acuity, lower-volume clinical programs, such as open-heart surgery and neurosurgery, and transporting patients from those programs to other system facilities. These changes ultimately improved clinical outcomes, given the greater expertise and higher volumes of the flagship programs. However, the physicians involved in those programs at the community hospital were suddenly left with fewer patients, and the community became concerned that the system was "gutting" its hospital.

A year into his role, the hospital president was called to an urgent meeting with the system CEO. In the meeting, the president was told that the hospital governing board, as a result of overwhelming staff and community feedback, was recommending he be removed from his position. Because the young president did not take the time to fully understand the organization's cultural dynamics and made drastic changes too quickly, he ultimately failed in a role for which he had the training and ability to succeed.

Be mindful: Assuming a new role is fraught with stress, challenges, and new expectations. Approaching the task with a structured onboarding plan can greatly enhance the chances of success.

MASTERING A NEW ROLE

There are few days in a leader's life as exciting and as frightening as the first day in a new position. Every promotional opportunity holds the promise of making a lasting impact on an organization and building a career legacy. At the same time, however, transition to a new role carries a risk of failure and career derailment, particularly if the onboarding process and early tenure in an organization are not carefully thought out. The higher the level of the new position, the greater the danger of failure.

People form impressions quickly, and these impressions, once established, can prove difficult to overcome. Executives' interactions with staff, their mannerisms, their style of dress, and the things they say (or, for that matter, don't say) in the first few months in a new role can make the difference between reaching their full potential and making an early exit. Staff, subordinates, and superiors intently scrutinize new executives' actions, inactions, and verbal and nonverbal communications. The protocol in this chapter, which is summarized in Exhibit 13.1, aims to help leaders step in with the "right foot."

EXHIBIT 13.1: Protocol for Success in a New Position

The following framework can provide guidance to executives when assuming a new role:

1. Look the part.
2. Plan for success.
3. Understand, then execute.
4. Be consistent.
5. Use the 1-1-3-7 guide.

Look the Part

Young executives are often told to dress for the role they aspire to hold, not necessarily the role they have today. This advice holds true for leaders at all levels, as appearance, mannerisms, grooming, and executive presence are key to establishing credibility with the people you hope to lead. The following actions can help executives come across as leaders:

- *Dress "interview ready."* Leaders should pay special attention to dress and hygiene, especially early in their tenure, because every person with whom they interact forms a first impression. These impressions can be long lasting and are often widely communicated (e.g., "The new boss looks really sharp," or "The new boss does not look very professional"). Always be well groomed, and wear simple, professional business attire to communicate that you care about your appearance and the way others perceive you.

- *Be on time.* Punctuality is a sign of respect, and tardiness signals to subordinates and superiors that you think your time is more valuable than theirs. Lateness can create the impression among staff that an executive feels "superior" to others and that the rules do not apply to her. If an executive is late to a meeting of superiors, such as board members, the tardiness may lead to perceptions that the executive is disorganized and cannot manage a schedule. "Fashionably late" should not be an inclination of a savvy leader.

- *Be visible.* A concerted curiosity surrounds any new boss, and executives new to their roles should take the time to walk through the organization on a daily basis, round with staff, and get to know their direct reports. Such interactions give leaders an air of approachability and help them craft the professional image they want others to hold.

Plan for Success

New executives should prepare a formal plan for the first several weeks in their new roles, and they should develop a personal leadership philosophy that can be succinctly, and frequently, communicated to the staff. A leadership philosophy statement—an expression of the leader's principles with memorable themes and phrases—can help make employees familiar with the new executive, his managerial style, and the values system by which he abides. Articulating a managerial style through a personal statement is similar to delivering a political message with a catchy, well-crafted slogan. Exhibit 13.2 provides some examples of leadership philosophy statements.

Additionally, Dickerson (2012) identified five sayings that all leaders should use frequently, and all five represent themes and statements especially appropriate for new leaders. The statements are shown in Exhibit 13.3.

EXHIBIT 13.2: Sample Leadership Philosophy Statements

"I was not hired here to come in and turn the organization around. You are already a very strong organization. I came here because I saw a great team that I could work with and help lead to the next level."

"My job as your new CEO is to help remove obstacles that get in the way of you doing your best work. I don't see myself as a micromanager but as a road clearer, helping set the direction but getting out of your way so that you can make the journey."

"Let's see what we can achieve together." —Microsoft CEO Satya Nadella (Microsoft News Center 2014)

EXHIBIT 13.3: Five Leadership Statements That Should Never Be Left Unsaid

"Great job."

"I believe in you."

"How can I help you?"

"I was wrong."

"Together we can."

Source: Dickerson (2012).

Understand, Then Execute

New leaders are often so eager to make their impression on an organization that they act without fully understanding the political, cultural, and interpersonal dynamics involved in their decisions. Barring a crisis, a leader should always take the appropriate amount of time to develop a thorough knowledge of the organization, and she should use this knowledge to act decisively. The following guidelines can assist in these matters:

- *Listen and learn.* In every organization, a new leader must deal with the expectations of others. The process of meeting with staff and exploring mutual expectations is vital during the first few months on the job, because it allows leaders to consider staff expectations as they map out their priorities for the organization. Many staff members are extremely cooperative and eager to teach new leaders about what they do.

- *Spend extra time at the office.* The amount of time a new executive spends on the job communicates his level of excitement and interest in the role. And frankly, the extra time may be necessary to gain foundational knowledge about the organization and its history, policies, stakeholder issues, and political dynamics.

- *Be alert and particularly attentive.* Possessing an auditor's curiosity is a healthy characteristic for all executives, but for new executives, it is an imperative. To gain a strong baseline understanding of the organization, you should thoughtfully question all activities that flow through and around your area of responsibility. Staff may initially resent some of this scrutiny, but you can reassure them by letting them know that such questioning is a key part of your orientation.

- *Be deliberate, but do not procrastinate.* New executives can postpone some decisions until they have gained a deeper understanding of the organizations, but other decisions cannot be put off. Even new leaders must act decisively when faced with vital decisions.

- *Spell out expectations.* New leaders should remember that staff may not intuitively understand what is expected of them and may be accustomed to a different leadership style. The leaders therefore should spell out their key expectations, describe their view of each direct report's role, and articulate the rationale behind their plans and actions. This advice applies both to day-to-day management functions and to the implementation of strategic changes.

Be Consistent

Leaders settling into new positions should strive to be the same person every day and not allow their demeanor and decision making to be influenced by emotions. Consistency, to a large extent, reflects a leader's emotional intelligence. Goleman (2004, 86) writes that "people who are in control of their feelings and impulses—that is, people who are reasonable—are able to create an environment of trust and fairness." Consistent behavior improves interpersonal relationships because staff members understand what to expect. The following guidelines can help new leaders demonstrate consistency.

- *Deliver on promises.* New leaders invariably receive lists of requests and suggestions from multiple stakeholder groups during their first weeks on the job. Leaders should be cautious about the commitments they make at this time, because failing to follow through on promises can lead to a swift loss of credibility. A written or electronic record of any commitments made can help keep this issue in check.

- *Display strengths.* Don't be afraid to show everyone why you were hired. If financial management is your primary language, then take the lead in the financial analysis of key initiatives. If you excel in building interpersonal relationships, focus on getting to know your employees. If strategy is your strong point, devote your time to that area. Whatever your specialty, ensure that your strengths shine through early in your tenure. Doing so can help you build a reputation of competence, knowledge, and experience.

- *Build interpersonal influence.* The ultimate success of any executive depends on her ability to leverage the relationships she builds to execute the plans she develops for the organization. As a leader, you sometimes will have to ask others to perform difficult tasks; their willingness to perform these tasks well may hinge on their relationships with you. Covey (2013) called this concept an "emotional bank account," in which leaders have to build equity with staff in order to make withdrawals at a future date.

Use the 1-1-3-7 Guide

A particularly useful tool for an executive in a new role is the 1-1-3-7 guide—so named because it represents actions that should occur on the first week, the first month, the third month, and the seventh month in a new role. The guide provides a framework to assist leaders in self-evaluation as they take on new responsibilities. The key steps are as follows:

- *Week 1.* At the end of the first week, new leaders should compile a list of five to ten key issues within the organization that will require their attention and five to ten leaders (formal or informal) with whom they will have to work effectively. The purpose of this list is to focus on present reality, to identify political dynamics, and to start recording ideas for necessary future changes. This list is a personal one and should be updated every few weeks.

- *Month 1.* As the first month concludes, new leaders should list five to eight expectations for their first six months and five to eight visible "early wins," or changes that could be implemented relatively easily and quickly. The expectations should be generic statements of behavior or descriptions of values (e.g., "doing things right the first time") that can be easily communicated to any group in the organization to underscore the type of behavior that will be valued under the new leadership. The ideas for change, on the other hand, should be specific and achievable; they should help the leader develop a reputation as an executive of action.

- *Month 3.* At the end of the third month, new leaders should update their list of key issues within the organization and present the issues to the organization's management team, or to the leadership team within the department. The third month is the optimal time for a summation because it allows the leader ample time to identify covert problems and to build enough personal equity with others to have relatively frank discussions regarding opportunities for improvement. These discussions represent the basis of ongoing dialogue to obtain input and form a strategic plan.

- *Month 7.* After the seventh month, leaders should have the framework for short-term actions that can be clearly articulated to the organization to address pressing concerns and for longer-term strategic initiatives that can guide organizational activities over the next several months.

The time frames for the 1-1-3-7 guide can vary. Some leaders prefer to think in terms of "the first 100 days," whereas others might choose longer periods. In some cases, an event such as a unionization campaign, an organizational financial crisis, or a significant physician issue might accelerate the timetable. Regardless of the increments chosen, the concepts remain the same. A clear framework and a thoughtful approach to planning the first few months in a new role will significantly increase the likelihood for success.

A final note is important: The 1-1-3-7 guide should be preserved as a written document that can be reviewed at a later date.

SELF-AWARENESS AND DERAILMENT

Many of the guidelines contained in this chapter—and elsewhere in the book, for that matter—involve a leader's ability to be self-aware and to avoid what management literature calls managerial "derailment." We refer readers to Chapter 17, which covers these topics in greater detail. The concepts of self-awareness and derailment are important for all leaders, but they are particularly applicable to leaders initially taking charge and assuming new positions.

SUMMARY

The field of healthcare management is littered with stories of leaders who experienced great success in one organization only to fail miserably as they made the transition to another. Similar stories of talented middle managers flaming out as they moved into broader leadership roles are also far too common. The leaders in these stories did not lose their skills or competencies in the new roles; often, they simply lacked planning and a thoughtful transition strategy. As healthcare undergoes fundamental changes, the knowledge required for leadership roles at all levels will evolve. The skills that made leaders successful in the first decade of their careers will likely be insufficient to ensure them sustained growth through retirement. Every new role provides leaders with valuable opportunities to hone their craft, but the stress of transition and the risk of failure are significant, especially in higher-level executive roles. Organizational politics, informal biases, fiscal concerns, and competitive threats constantly pressure leaders to take swift action as they assume new positions. If leaders operate in a vacuum and fail to take into account cultural dynamics and the issues facing the organization, their actions may not produce optimal outcomes. The protocol in this chapter provides a framework for leaders in new leadership roles and aims to enhance their chances for sustained success.

GUEST COMMENTARY: JOHN "JACK" R. JANOSO, JR.

Achieving early adoption and credible acceptance in a new organization requires a calculated approach with as much strategy and forethought as the organization's business plan. The potential for a good fit actually begins in the evaluative phase of the hiring or promotion process, where both the new executive and the organization's incumbent leaders must gain insight into synergy of purpose, managerial style, and fundamental relationship building— elements that can quickly impact the success or failure of the business strategy and objectives. Harbored anger and disenfranchisement can easily derail the best of intentions if there is a mismatch in expectations or early difficulty in establishing trust with key organizational stakeholders.

Having recently made a transition as the new CEO of a successful organization, I have found that the abilities to learn on the job, to keep one's "mouth shut and ears open," and to act like a "guest" rather than a new "owner"

(continued)

(continued from previous page)

helped set a tone of thoughtful respect and humility with important and influential members of the organization. This tone was intentional and critical, because much of my early evaluation as a new leader came from these stakeholders and not from announcements or one-on-one discussions. I spent significant time learning about the issues and concerns of the organization while formulating a plan to address the most critical needs. As this "break-in" period was proceeding, the natural tendency was to compare and contrast my leadership style with that of the previous CEO, and some people tested to see how far I could be pressed on personal issues and agendas. This period presented my greatest opportunity to demonstrate leadership as well as a new vision, relationship, and cultural philosophy, centered around the strengths of the organization. It also presented me an opportunity to acknowledge the prior failures of management but to refuse the burdens of "old baggage" and issues that were no longer relevant. Deliberate and strategic overcommunication was an important credibility-building technique that, when coupled with absolute transparency, left little room for misinterpretation. Being sensitive and self-aware also helped considerably, as I would continually ask for, and provide, immediate and direct feedback to all constituents. Changes have been made—in some cases, difficult ones—but there has been full disclosure as to why these changes have been necessary. The most important foundation for success has been the articulation of our new organizational culture and values. They have been thoughtfully crafted and personally

(continued)

(continued from previous page)

communicated by myself as CEO to each member of the organization.

It has been encouraging and rewarding to see the transformation of the culture take hold and the staff begin to engage. Change can be hard to fathom, but stagnation and irrelevance are death sentences to community health organizations. A new CEO should bring change but make haste carefully and deliberately.

John "Jack" R. Janoso, Jr.
President and CEO, Fairfield Medical Center
Lancaster, Ohio

REFLECTIVE QUESTIONS

1. Reflect on the vignette at the beginning of the chapter. What could this new president have done to make his transition into the new organization more successful?

2. Even if you have been in your current leadership role for some time, you should always be evolving as a leader to better serve your staff. Starting today, consider following a 1-1-3-7 guideline to formalize your departmental or organizational strategy over the coming months.

RESOURCES AND EXERCISES FOR LEADERSHIP DEVELOPMENT

1. Do you have a leadership theme or "mantra"? What do you stand for? Can your fundamental beliefs about leadership be fit within a two-minute "elevator speech"?

2. So many leaders feel great pressure to deliver quick results early in their tenure in new positions. Research this tendency and outline the reasons for it. Begin with a review of an excellent article from the *Harvard Business Review*, "The Quick Wins Paradox" (https://hbr.org/2009/01/the-quick-wins-paradox).

3. When starting a new leadership role, be sure to have an outside confidante who provides thoughts about how you are doing early in the onboarding process.

4. Investigate the practice of onboarding.

REFERENCES

Covey, S. R. 2013. *The 7 Habits of Highly Effective People: Powerful Lessons in Personal Change*, 25th anniversary ed. New York: Simon and Schuster.

Dickerson, D. 2012. "5 Leadership Statements That Should Never Be Left Unsaid." *International Business Times.* Published October 12. www.ibtimes.com/exnet/5-leadership-statements-should-never-be-left-unsaid-853244.

Goleman, D. 2004. "What Makes a Leader?" *Harvard Business Review* 82 (1): 82–91.

Microsoft News Center. 2014. "Satya Nadella Email to Employees: RE: Grace Hopper Conference." Published October 9. http://news.microsoft.com/2014/10/09/satya-nadella-email-to-employees-re-grace-hopper-conference/.

Watkins, M. 2003. *The First 90 Days: Critical Success Strategies for New Leaders at All Levels*. Boston: Harvard Business School Press.

CHAPTER 14

The Office

Like traffic signals and road maps, office protocol keeps us from crashing into one another, from hurting colleagues' feelings, or from damaging a firm's reputation.

—Amy Vanderbilt

Guide to Reader

The office setting has become a focus of pop culture, with cartoons such as *Dilbert* and television shows such as *The Office*. Unfortunately, many portrayals of the office setting, though humorous, signal the fact that behavior in this setting is often less than proper. Much of this chapter focuses on issues of common courtesy and demeanor in the work setting—the setting in which leaders spend the most time, and where they often display the most improper conduct.

Small Errors with Large Implications

A well-respected CEO had a reputation as a keenly adept businessman with an uncanny knack for evaluating complex strategic situations and determining the appropriate course of action to ensure the organization's ongoing success. During his 15 years at the helm of a large integrated healthcare delivery system, he had received national acclaim as an innovative leader, and the facilities under his authority were among the best in the country in terms of patient outcomes, quality, and financial performance.

Because he had worked his way up from a line-manager position, the CEO also prided himself on staying true to his "everyman" roots. He felt the key to remaining connected to the operations of the health system was to develop personal and informal relationships with the members of his office staff and with subordinate executives. Problems developed, however, when these relationships and the CEO's behavior started bordering on unprofessional and violated the fundamentals of good office etiquette.

A gregarious person by nature, the CEO was known to crack jokes with his staff without regard for who might be within earshot. On occasion, staff members who overheard jokes with slightly sexual undertones were offended.

The CEO also believed in the power of "personal touch" to create connections with his staff. He felt that the best way to let people know he cared about them was to give them a pat on the back or even a hug. Several individuals on his team, however, felt this contact was disrespectful and outside the bounds of appropriate executive behavior.

(continued)

(continued from previous page)

Finally, having been raised in the South, the CEO felt that referring to members of the office support staff with informal terms of endearment such as "sweetie" or "honey" was perfectly acceptable. He relied on such terms in part because he had a difficult time recalling names, and he feared that asking staff members to remind him of their names would make him appear uncaring. One office staff member complained to her peers that the CEO had been calling her by the wrong name for over a year, and now she just smiled and responded to the incorrect salutation every time he walked by.

Eventually, complaints to human resources, the frequent turnover of support staff in the CEO office, and a mounting number of anonymous calls to the hospital compliance hotline caused the board of trustees to take notice. When the board informed the CEO of the themes that were emerging around his lack of workplace manners, he was both surprised and reflective. He apologized to his team and volunteered for additional training on office etiquette. A year later, his behavior was much improved, as was the morale of those in the executive office.

Be mindful: As healthcare leaders, we often spend more time in the office than we do with our families. We should therefore demonstrate the same sense of ownership and pride in our work environment as we do with our home.

APPROPRIATE OFFICE ETIQUETTE

Taken individually, the lapses in office protocol by the CEO in the vignette might seem minor, but an accumulation of small slip-ups can create deep resentment and lead to significant reductions in team effectiveness. Executives set the tone for office culture, and in many ways the office becomes a physical extension of the executive. The actions of leaders are under great scrutiny and have a lasting impact on staff behavior and morale.

Perceptions of the executive suite as an "ivory tower" can arouse feelings of curiosity, fear, and envy among frontline staff. If a CEO spends her day working behind closed doors, the rest of the staff might feel that she does not value an open environment and dislikes informal interaction and "hallway" conversation. Likewise, if a vice president constantly witnesses his peer executives working on their smartphones and iPads during meetings, he is likely to adopt that behavior himself, even if it is rude to other attendees. Seemingly minor details such as eating strong-smelling food in close proximity to others, not cleaning up after oneself in the office kitchen, speaking loudly, and interrupting others in an open work environment can all contribute to a toxic office culture.

Over the years, the strict formality of many executive suites has loosened and given way to a more relaxed setting with increased cultural openness. This transition has led to stronger leader–staff relationships in many organizations, but it also carries a risk. Excessive informality can translate into complacency, carelessness, and poor office etiquette, and overly familiar executives can behave, perhaps unintentionally, in ways that others perceive as inappropriate or rude. According to Pearson and Porath (2009), 96 percent of American workers experience rude behavior at work, and 48 percent say it occurs at least once per week. Moreover, nearly half the workers who were treated rudely reported that they intentionally decreased their productivity as a result of the poor work environment. It is a fact: Even minor lapses in manners have lasting negative impacts on organizations.

Some leaders profess to not play "office politics." Many subscribe to the viewpoint of Graham (1998), who links office politics with "hypocrisy, secrecy, deal making, rumors, power brokers, self-interest, image-building, self-promotion, and cliques." However, to a certain extent, office politics is unavoidable. Cheok (2015) writes that, at its most basic level, "office politics is simply about the differences between people at work. . . . It all goes down to human communications and relationships." Leaders spend much of their work time inside the C-suite offices, and they must learn to navigate these tricky waters.

Most inappropriate office behavior results from lack of self-awareness rather than a true intention to offend others. The protocol presented here, and summarized in Exhibit 14.1, will help leaders remain attentive to their behavior, carry out professional interactions in the office, and strike the right balance between formality and familiarity.

EXHIBIT 14.1: Protocol for Appropriate Office Etiquette

The following framework can help leaders manage their interactions in the office setting:

1. Know and respect the culture.
2. Keep personal and professional lives separate.
3. View your actions through the eyes of others.
4. Develop an attention to details.
5. Be professionally sociable.
6. Don't get too comfortable.

Know and Respect the Culture

Every office setting has an established culture, or a set of behavioral norms that have developed and been reinforced over time. The culture defines what behavior is acceptable in the eyes of the people working in the office, as well as how those people expect to be treated by others. The norms can be as simple as placing one's name on personal food in the break-room refrigerator or as complex as a formal communication style preferred among the executive staff. Any deviation from these accepted behaviors, intentional or not, can be considered rude and offensive. Absent a sound understanding of the office culture, leaders should err on the side of conservatism and professionalism. This advice is especially true early in one's tenure. The following actions can assist in this regard:

- *Participate in—and respect—appropriate office traditions.* Departments, teams, and office staff develop traditions that strengthen their work dynamics and personal camaraderie. Leaders should take part in these practices, or at least respect them if they are not invited to join. For example, if an office tradition involves a weekly potluck lunch every Friday, the executive should ask the coordinator what she can bring to support the initiative. If an executive encounters an office practice that is not appropriate for the work setting, he should provide a detailed rationale to the staff before ending or changing it.

- *Be cautious with humor.* An office is fundamentally a serious place: It exists for work to be accomplished. The office is not a place for executives with comedic career aspirations to try out new jokes. By their nature, healthcare organizations have individuals from all walks of life, and what is humorous to one group might be offensive to another. Often, anecdotes intended to lighten the mood actually make people uncomfortable and decrease productivity and morale.

Keep Personal and Professional Lives Separate

Leaders and their staffs work closely together, both literally and figuratively. This closeness leads to friendships, and many friendships grow to the point that executives, staff members, and their families socialize together outside of the work environment. Such friendships can be a strong cog in the machinery of team building, but they can also be harmful if team members become too comfortable with one another and carry too much informality back into the workplace. An overly relaxed atmosphere can be counterproductive and disruptive, especially when the team has to deal with difficult issues. The following guidelines can help leaders draw appropriate boundaries between their personal and professional lives:

- *Be mindful of power.* Executives should realize that their formal power in an organization has the potential to intimidate others, and they should be conscious of how their power might affect interactions. For example, a staff member might be placed in an awkward position if she is asked to buy fundraising tickets from an executive's child. Additionally, executives should not ask support staff to do personal favors that are not related to their jobs (e.g., purchasing personal birthday gifts, placing personal calls for the executive).

- *Keep conversations professional.* Executives should keep discussions of personal affairs out of the office. Lighthearted exchanges about family or personal interests may help team members get to know one another, but more serious and intimate issues, such as marital and financial problems, should be avoided. Change the subject if you feel you need to extricate yourself from such a discussion.

- *Decorate the office appropriately.* Customizing the office to reflect one's personal style is permissible, but doing so should not conflict with the general décor of the organization or be distracting to others.

- *Never borrow money from coworkers.* Loans between coworkers are dangerous because they put both the lender and the borrower in uncomfortable positions. Borrowing may suggest that staff members trust and feel at ease with one another, but it can also be a sign of future unrest.

View Your Actions Through the Eyes of Others

Remember that the executive office serves as a visible representation of the organization as a whole and that you, as a leader, set the tone for how the office culture evolves. Your own actions communicate to the staff what behaviors are expected and rewarded. The following tactics can help you send the "right" message:

- *Ensure the physical appropriateness of the office.* Factors such as the neatness of the office and the respect and courtesy shown by the staff send a strong message about the professionalism of an organization. If the office is cluttered and staff members are eating at their desks with food odors permeating the suite, people will receive an inappropriate message.

- *Show common courtesy.* Executives can often fall into a habit of being informal with team members, particularly if they have been working together for a long time. Even routine interpersonal exchanges, however, should be courteous. Team members should understand that they are not taken for granted.

- *Do not treat support staff as servants.* Running personal errands for the executive, buying and wrapping gifts for the executive's spouse, and handling chores for family members are not appropriate tasks for an administrative assistant. Support staff are in the office to help facilitate professional success, not to be your personal concierge.

- *Share information.* Leaders should inform colleagues and support staff of the rationale behind major decisions, and they should openly discuss the direction the organization is taking. Keeping others "in the know" builds a stronger and better aligned team.

- *Clarify expectations.* In team interactions, the executive should speak openly about expectations such as the necessity to work over a long weekend, the importance of confidentiality, or the best way to work together. Clarifying key issues up front will reduce the risk of misunderstandings later.

Develop an Attention to Details

Executives can improve the personal impressions they make and the overall sense of professionalism in the office by paying attention to seemingly minor details in their interactions. Indeed, these "little things" can often make or break simple interactions. Consider these suggestions:

- If you are holding a drink, keep it in your left hand so that the right hand is dry and free to shake hands (this advice applies outside the office at cocktail parties and receptions).
- If you are handed a business card, respectfully look at the details of the card before placing it in your pocket.
- Work diligently to know the names of the people with whom you work, as well as the names of their spouses and children. Populate your calendar with important dates for people in the executive office so that you can personally reach out to them.
- If you are hosting an event, arrive early, stay late, and mingle with everyone at the party, especially people whom you do not already know. If necessary, skip dessert so that you have time to meet everyone. One CEO remarked, "these social events are often the most important places where I can make strong personal impressions—I don't go to 'party,' I go to work."

Be Professionally Sociable

Executives live exceptionally social lives, with receptions, lunches, and dinners thrown by a multitude of hosts for a multitude of reasons. Leaders in social settings must represent their organization well, and they should use socializing opportunities to get to know peers and employees, to make business connections, and to garner support. The following guidelines can help leaders mix socially in a professional manner:

- *Be gracious.* Leaders hosting a lunch or dinner should make all the necessary arrangements in advance. They should ensure a private and comfortable seating arrangement and let the server know who will be receiving the check. Restaurants with which the host is already familiar are the safest choices. The host should arrive early and escort guests to the table.
- *Observe proper decorum.* During a business lunch or dinner, the focus should be on the business agenda. Excessive drinking, overly personal or unprofessional dialogue, or other rude behavior should be avoided.
- *Respect others' time.* Early in a lunch or dinner, the host should find out if any of the other individuals have time constraints. If time is a factor, move into the business discussions shortly after drinks have arrived.

Don't Get Too Comfortable

Let's face it: Society in many ways has become less formal and more laid-back, as the informality associated with "casual Fridays" has spread into other aspects of workplace culture. Fischer (2015) writes, "Americans have become strikingly informal: we deviate from convention more than we used to, and the conventions we do observe entail less deference to institutions such as churches and statuses such as advanced age." He goes on to state that, as a society, Americans have "sought to discard the falsity of custom in preference for an 'authentic' self." Leaders should be aware that this trend carries an inherent risk, and they should always hold themselves to a higher standard.

Leaders should carefully observe office protocols and be on guard against becoming too casual, too informal, or too relaxed. The office should be viewed first and foremost as a serious place where work is done; by staying true to that principle, leaders can keep casual Fridays from disrupting their careers. To maintain perspective, consider the advice of the *Wall Street Journal* (2009), which urges leaders to ponder the following questions when dealing with office politics: "What are the core values and how are they enacted? Are short- or long-term results more valued? How are decisions made? How much risk is tolerated?"

SUMMARY

The executive office is a microcosm of the organization as a whole. The culture and behaviors demonstrated by executives set a benchmark that others within the organization will observe and emulate. Executive leaders must establish the appropriate tone of professionalism through their words and actions while still creating an open environment in which people are excited to work. Such a balance can be difficult to maintain, but the protocol described in this chapter can assist in that regard.

GUEST COMMENTARY: MICHELLE TAYLOR SMITH

Do You Hear What I See?

I was waiting for the start of my first executive leadership meeting since my promotion. While waiting, I took note of the large oval-shaped table and turned my attention to the layout of the room. I noticed there were no chairs on the periphery of the room, away from the large oval table. This detail may not have been important to many, but to me it spoke volumes. The fact that all chairs were positioned at the oval table said to me that this was an organization that embraced inclusion. In that moment, the aesthetic proxemics I observed set the tone for the interpersonal relationship I expected and ultimately would experience with the leadership of the organization (Hall 1963).

Expounding on Relationships as the Basis of Leadership

As important as the Industrial Revolution was to the evolution of task orientation in the workplace, equally important were the Hawthorne Studies, conducted from 1927 to 1932, in examining the workplace's human element. However, it has taken some time for leadership in organizations to "get it" and understand the critical need for "soft skills." The reasons soft skills and interpersonal relationships have become so important involve a wide variety of factors:

- In 2015, millennials (generation Y) were predicted to become the largest percentage of the workforce for the first time.

(continued)

(continued from previous page)

- The current era is the first time in American history that we have had *four* different generations working side by side in the workplace.

- Organizational infrastructures now mandate teams and departments.

- Interpersonal skills are "hardwired" in the neuronal pathways of the cerebral cortex. Behavior patterns are physically established at the brain cell level. At some point, a behavior is repeated often enough that neurons grow dendrites that reach out to other neurons to establish the connections needed to make a behavior pattern automatic. Any new pattern—even one that makes sense, even one that is desired and expected— will seem extremely awkward.

- The brain processes verbal and nonverbal communication at the same time and notices when people's words don't match their body language. Much of our nonverbal communication is unconscious. Nonverbal communication is not just something we do to show how we are feeling; we also depend on our interpretations of it when we interact.

Woven Threads

While assessing the importance of soft skills and interpersonal relationships in the workplace, we must recognize that all individuals come to organizations with their skill set well ingrained. Behavior modification takes time and reinforcement, and the differences that exist

(continued)

(continued from previous page)

across multiple generations can complicate matters—it's a recipe that necessitates nurturing of the desired skill set.

Because most graduate schools don't teach how to cultivate soft skills, organizations and leaders alike are being taken to task to instill these skills into the fabric of the organizational culture. Honing these skills can help organizations create a competitive advantage and distinguish them from being cookie-cutter look-alikes (Nicolaides 2014).

As previously stated, leadership is a complex task that relies on the engagement and actions of others for success. All leaders should ensure that their leadership voice matches their leadership action. Personally, I envision the day when everyone will have the opportunity to experience what I did at my very first executive-level meeting. Did I hear what I saw? The response will be a resounding YES!

Michelle Taylor Smith, MSN, RN, NE-BC, FACHE
Vice President, Patient Care Services/Chief Nursing Office
Greenville Hospital System
Greenville, South Carolina

REFLECTIVE QUESTIONS

1. What are some activities that have become office traditions in your work environment? Do they set the appropriate tone of professionalism?

2. Reflect on how you personally interact with your coworkers and support staff. How might the protocol in this chapter improve the balance between formality and familiarity?

RESOURCES AND EXERCISES FOR LEADERSHIP DEVELOPMENT

1. Browse the numerous *Dilbert* cartoons that are available online (www.dilbert.com), and find five or six that depict a situation that resembles one of your own real-life experiences.

2. Review these two excellent articles dealing with office politics:

    Nemko, M. 2015. "Win at Office Politics Without Selling Your Soul." Monster. Accessed September 21. http://career-advice.monster.com/in-the-office /workplace-issues/win-at-office-politics/article.aspx.

    Reardon, K. K. 2015. "Office Politics Isn't Something You Can Sit Out." *Harvard Business Review*. Published January 12. https://hbr.org/2015/01 /office-politics-isnt-something-you-can-sit-out.

3. Secure and read a comprehensive book on etiquette and manners. *The Amy Vanderbilt Complete Book of Etiquette, 50th Anniversary Edition* (Doubleday, 1995) is excellent, as is *Emily Post's The Etiquette Advantage in Business: Personal Skills for Professional Success,* second edition (William Morrow Publishing, 2005).

4. Consider the dangers of casual dress, and review some guides to proper business dress. Some of the better ones are provided by Salisbury University (www.salisbury .edu/careerservices/students/Interviews/Dress.html), the Marine Corps (www.hqmc.marines.mil/Portals/133 /Docs/MCIA%20Dress%20Code.pdf), Virginia Tech (www .career.vt.edu/JobSearchGuide/BusinessCasualAttire.html), and the Society for Human Resource Management (www .shrm.org/templatestools/samples/policies/pages /businessandcasualattirepolicy.aspx).

REFERENCES

Cheok, L. 2015. "7 Habits To Win In Office Politics." *Lifehack*, 2015. Accessed April 11. www.lifehack.org/articles/work /7-habits-to-win-in-office-politics.html.

Fischer, C. S. 2015. "Dressing Down." *Boston Review*. Published February 16. http://bostonreview.net/claude-fischer-made -america-dressing-down.

Graham, G. 1998. "Eliminate Office Politics and End Many Problems in Companies." *Wichita Business Journal*. Published February 8. www.bizjournals.com/wichita/stories/1998/02/09/news column4.html.

Hall, E. T. 1963. "A System for the Notation of Proxemic Behavior." *American Anthropologist* 65 (5): 1003–1026.

Nicolaides, C. 2014. "Focus on Soft Skills: A Leadership Wake-Up Call." Business Know-How. Accessed December 19. www .businessknowhow.com/growth/softskills.htm.

Pearson, C., and C. Porath. 2009. *The Cost of Bad Behavior: How Incivility Is Damaging Your Business and What to Do About It.* New York: Penguin Group.

Wall Street Journal. 2009. "How to Handle Office Politics." Published May 8. http://guides.wsj.com/careers/how-to -overcome-career-obstacles/how-to-handle-office-politics/tab /print/.

CHAPTER 15

Ethnic and Gender Diversity

Strength lies in differences, not in similarities.

—Stephen Covey

Guide to Reader

The ability to work effectively with diversity is a key element of any leader's skill set, and it begins with having the proper attitude and beliefs. Leaders must embrace diversity and differences—not just because doing so is mandated, but because it is natural. The most effective leaders work effortlessly with diverse groups and, frankly, rarely highlight individual differences other than those of critical leadership competencies. The protocols described in this chapter should not only be learned; they should become second nature.

A Flawed Melting Pot

A small suburban hospital was the outermost healthcare provider in a large metropolitan area, and it served patients both from the immediate community and from the surrounding rural areas. The administrative team of the hospital took great pride in developing strong clinical programs that were not typical of a facility of its size. The administration successfully developed higher-end programs—such as open heart services, cancer care, and a neonatal intensive care unit—to provide alternatives to patients who in the past had to drive an hour or longer into sprawling urban medical campuses to obtain such services. The community embraced the rapidly evolving capabilities of the hospital, and the facility was poised for tremendous growth in the future.

Despite the hospital's success and positive reputation in the community, the administrative team became concerned that staff turnover was rising every year. The facility had always prided itself on staff retention—a priority reflected by the fact that the C-suite executives had all been with the organization for more than 10 years. But some recent discontent had surfaced, especially among younger staff, and overall turnover numbers were approaching 35 percent annually. Even more concerning was the feedback received in exit interviews. The key theme of the feedback was a perception that the organization and its leadership did not value diversity.

The surrounding community had been largely Caucasian for much of the hospital's history, but over the past five years, a number of Hispanic and African-American families had

(continued)

(continued from previous page)

moved to the area. The administrative team consisted entirely of white male executives, but the team had publicly stated that the organizational culture valued diversity. Prompted by the staff feedback, hospital leadership brought in an outside consultant to help assess the issues and to provide recommendations on how to reverse the negative sentiments.

When the consultant arrived, the opportunities for improvement were glaring. She immediately noticed that, even though the hospital's patient population had become nearly 30 percent Hispanic, the hospital had no bilingual directional signs and offered only limited access to interpretive services. The consultant also noted that, although the hospital had begun hiring a more diverse workforce, the middle management had very few minority or female leaders among its ranks, and the senior leadership had none.

In essence, the C-suite executives had seen the community change around them but did little to modify the care environment to make it more welcoming to the community. Moreover, although the leaders had worked to fill the talent pipeline with a more diverse group of employees, they had failed to actively cultivate this pipeline; as a result, high-potential individuals with ethnic or gender backgrounds different from those of the senior leadership team assumed that they had no path for continued growth and chose to leave. The C-suite leaders may have philosophically espoused a desire for enhanced diversity, but in their actions, they did little to ensure that diversity became a key organizational priority.

(continued)

(continued from previous page)

Be mindful: The lens through which we see our organizations is crafted by our own unique backgrounds and life experiences. Embracing diversity in the workplace creates a rich tapestry of opinions that can prevent a leadership team from becoming myopic in its decision making.

A CHANGING WORKFORCE

To start, consider the following:

- The percentage of Americans identifying themselves as black, Hispanic, Asian, or "other" increased from just 15 percent of the population in 1960 to 36 percent in 2010 (Taylor 2014).
- The US Census Bureau began collecting detailed data on multiracial people in 2000, when it first allowed respondents to select more than one race. That year, "6.8 million people chose to do so. Ten years later that number jumped by 32 percent, making it one of the fastest growing categories" (Funderburg 2013).
- "Census data tell us that by 2050 there will be no racial or ethnic majority in our country. Further, between 2000 and 2050 new immigrants and their children will account for 83 percent of the growth in the working-age population" (Burns, Barton, and Kerby 2012).
- Gin (2013) writes: "We are so much more than color, race, ethnicity, culture and traditions. Diversity in the 21st century needs to recognize age, gender, sexual orientation, economic condition and lifestyle. But, we also should acknowledge and embrace differing perspectives as a core element of diversity."

Few world events have represented such major strides toward gender and racial equality in leadership as the 2008 election for president of the United States. Ever since the country was founded, the roles of president and vice president had been held by Caucasian males, but the 2008 campaign showed an unprecedented diversity in its set of candidates. The Democratic primary was a hard-fought battle between two US senators, one an African American and the other a female. Though Hillary Clinton fell short of breaking what she termed "the highest glass ceiling," she made significant cracks in it by garnering 18 million votes. Meanwhile, the Republican ticket had its own female candidate, Alaska governor Sarah Palin, who became the first female vice presidential candidate on a major-party ticket in more than 30 years. The remarkable contest culminated with the election of Barack Obama as the country's first African-American commander-in-chief. Today, a similar shift toward diversity in leadership can be seen in healthcare: The stakes may not be as high as in the Oval Office, but a variety of studies indicate that hospital C-suites—once dominated by white male professionals—are becoming much more reflective of the population as a whole.

Studies by the American College of Healthcare Executives (ACHE) have identified a number of trends in the makeup of healthcare leadership. A 2012 survey on the career advancement of males and females found that 11 percent of women in healthcare leadership attain the title of CEO during the course of their careers (ACHE 2012). The same study indicated that women make up a majority of senior leadership roles in specialized areas such as planning, marketing, and quality assurance. In 2008, ACHE and the National Association of Health Services Executives revisited an earlier study, titled *A Racial/Ethnic Comparison of Career Attainment in Healthcare Management*, with the support of the Asian Health Care Leaders Association, the Institute for Diversity in Health Management, and the National Forum for Latino Healthcare Executives. The study surveyed a broad base of members from the organizations' databases and yielded valuable information about the changing backgrounds of healthcare leaders. In particular, the study reported that the following percentages from various groups held senior leadership positions such as CEO or COO/senior vice president (ACHE et al. 2008):

- 20 percent of African-American female respondents
- 39 percent of African-American male respondents
- 37 percent of Hispanic female respondents
- 43 percent of Hispanic male respondents
- 21 percent of Asian female respondents
- 22 percent of Asian male respondents
- 31 percent of white female respondents
- 56 percent of white male respondents

These statistics reflect major demographic shifts within healthcare organizations and in the communities they serve, and they show progress in terms of leadership diversity. Still, much work remains to be done. Additional findings from the same study include the following (ACHE et al. 2008):

- Women still achieve CEO positions in the healthcare industry at about half the rate of their male counterparts, and women are less likely than men to report a satisfactory work–life balance.
- Women and nonwhite male executives still report being compensated at a rate 20 to 30 percent less than their white male counterparts for similar roles.
- More than 50 percent of African-American respondents, 27 percent of Hispanic respondents, and 31 percent of Asian respondents report that they have been negatively affected by racial or ethnic discrimination in their careers.

Concerns about inequality and discrimination were further highlighted by a 2014 ACHE survey involving race relations in the workplace. As shown in Exhibit 15.1, minority respondents were significantly less likely than white respondents to perceive their organizations' race relations as "good" (ACHE 2015).

Even as leadership teams increasingly emphasize multiculturalism and verbally commit to diversity, further advancements in *action* are needed to close the gaps noted in these studies. In the years ahead, the ability of healthcare leaders to manage and meet

EXHIBIT 15.1: Percent Agreeing with Statements About Organizational Race Relations

Statement	Percent Agreeing with Statement			
	Asian	Black	Hispanic	White
Race relations in my organization are good.*	76%	53%	76%	83%
Minority managers usually have to be more qualified than others to get ahead in my organization.*	29%	69%	22%	6%
The quality of relationships between minority and white managers here could be improved.*	28%	52%	24%	17%
The quality of relationships between minorities from different racial/ethnic groups could be improved here.*	38%	52%	31%	22%
A greater effort should be made in my organization to increase the percentage of racial/ethnic minorities in senior healthcare management positions.*	59%	81%	53%	40%

* Differences by race/ethnicity statistically significant at $p < .05$

Source: Reprinted with permission from *Chief Executive Officer* newsletter, American College of Healthcare Executives (2015).

the needs of an increasingly diverse workforce will be critical, and an organization that truly embraces diversity in its leadership ranks will have a sustainable competitive advantage among its peers.

The foundation for the protocols in this chapter is respect. Respect both drives and is driven by curiosity about people who come from different cultures, who practice different traditions, who subscribe to different beliefs, or who simply vary in physical appearance. Respect cannot be faked or given superficially. A leader who pretends to embrace diversity in words but does not demonstrate this commitment in action will quickly have his disingenuousness exposed, which can be extremely harmful to an individual's career and equally disastrous for an organization. Miller and Katz (2002, ix) make the point rather directly: "Diversity and inclusion must be at the core of an organization's culture. There is no such thing as a successful 'get by' diversity strategy."

ENHANCING RACIAL, ETHNIC, AND CULTURAL DIVERSITY

Respect encourages the treatment of people as individuals and discourages easy belief in stereotypes. It also embraces the concept of inclusiveness. Inclusiveness requires that a person or an organization move well beyond simply accepting people who are different; it requires genuine action to incorporate into the culture a welcoming attitude toward all viewpoints and perspectives. In reality, the concept of inclusiveness describes a journey rather than a final destination. Inclusiveness means that the culture strives to be open, transparent, and considerate of all. The following protocol, which is summarized in Exhibit 15.2, will assist leaders in promoting respect and inclusiveness for those of different racial, ethnic, and cultural backgrounds.

The following framework can provide guidance to leaders seeking to enhance racial, ethnic, and cultural diversity:

1. Embrace diversity as an organizational priority.
2. Assemble a diverse governance structure.
3. Celebrate other cultures.
4. Grow diverse talent.

Embrace Diversity as an Organizational Priority

Executive leaders set the agenda for change within their organizations, and their visible commitment to diversity is essential for overcoming inertia and achieving progress. Leaders should include diversity in key organizational documents such as the vision statement, articulate specific diversity-related goals in the strategic plan, and use personal influence to motivate others toward the idea of a more diverse organization. Organizations that have been most successful in creating a multicultural environment have made diversity a key organizational priority that personally involves the entire executive team, starting with the CEO. Some proactive steps that an organization can take include the following:

- *Promote diversity.* All executives should talk about diversity within their own teams and educate staff about its importance. Human resources executives should be especially active advocates, keeping the executive team aware of diversity issues in the workforce and speaking up in favor of programs that promote the advancement of minority groups through hiring, training, and education.
- *Create an open dialogue.* Racial tensions and sociopolitical issues between groups can be uncomfortable topics, and in many organizations they are not openly discussed. As a result, many problems are not properly confronted and

resolved but rather "swept under the rug." Prejudice is divisive, and it is largely based on misperception and fear. A candid dialogue and a commitment to ongoing training on diversity issues can raise awareness of hidden biases and encourage true acceptance rather than quiet tolerance.

- *Require diversity in searches for key leadership positions.* Many organizations require that a minority candidate be included on the "short list" when recruiting for any senior-level position, and such requirements have been associated with greater job satisfaction among leaders of diverse backgrounds. Most organizations have focused their efforts on growing diverse talent in entry-level leadership roles and providing a clear path for advancement to diverse leaders entering the talent pipeline. Providing minority candidates with chances to interview can go a long way in helping them develop.

Assemble a Diverse Governance Structure

An organization's governing board should mirror the community it serves and have fair representation in its views and decisions. Executives therefore must recruit board members with backgrounds similar to those of the organization's service population. Some organizations have a governing board subcommittee dedicated solely to diversity enhancement or a chief diversity officer (CDO) who oversees diversity-related strategic goals.

Celebrate Other Cultures

An organization-wide celebration of diversity can contribute greatly to the environment of acceptance. For instance, "theme days"—in which a specific culture's food, art, music, and literature are celebrated in a public gathering area, such as the cafeteria—can help educate staff and provide a visible representation of the leadership team's commitment to a multicultural approach. Special holidays and month-long observances—such as Black History Month, Chinese New Year, and Cinco de Mayo—should be recognized, with specific events receiving special emphasis based on the makeup and interests of your employee and patient populations. Inviting employees to share information about their cultures is another way to promote understanding. For instance, one medical laboratory with a particularly diverse workforce placed a map of the world on the break-room wall and marked each country from which an employee hailed. The lab went on to have potluck lunches in which employees brought dishes from their home countries and provided background about their traditions.

Grow Diverse Talent

The most effective and lasting way to improve leadership diversity is to create a pipeline of talented individuals from various backgrounds. Because some cultures may not actively encourage young people to explore careers in healthcare leadership, people already in the profession can serve as the best ambassadors. Consider the following actions:

- *Participate in community programs that enhance diversity.* Consider an "adopt-a-school" program in which the organization uses its resources and staff volunteers to provide training, workshops, or mentoring to minority students who have expressed an interest in the healthcare professions.
- *Use administrative residencies and fellowships to create a diversity pipeline.* In the diversity study described earlier in the chapter, researchers found that, among certain minority groups, more than half the students who completed residencies were eventually hired by their

organizations, and an even higher percentage of those who completed postgraduate fellowships remained as members of the leadership team (ACHE et al. 2008). Such programs represent not only a way for executives to share their expertise with the next generation of healthcare leaders but also a means to attract qualified minority candidates.

- *Provide formal mentoring to promote diversity.* Many individuals who achieve success as leaders in healthcare do so in part because of mentorship arrangements, in which experienced leaders devote their personal time to help newer leaders build their skill sets. However, connecting with a willing mentor can be challenging, especially if the new leader differs culturally from members of the current executive team. Organizations can help break down these potential barriers by establishing a formal mentoring program for emerging talent from diverse backgrounds.

ENHANCING GENDER DIVERSITY

The same respect and inclusiveness directed toward people of different racial, ethnic, and cultural backgrounds should be applied to employees of different genders. At the same time, leaders should be aware of additional considerations that apply specifically to the aim of gender equality in the workplace. The following protocol, summarized in Exhibit 15.3, can help ensure healthy gender diversity and an appropriate work environment for both male and female employees:

EXHIBIT 15.3: Protocol for Enhancing Gender Diversity

The following framework can help promote the success of female executives in an organization:

1. Establish a harassment-free workplace.
2. Ensure pay and advancement equity.
3. Support balance between work and family commitments.

Establish a Harassment-Free Workplace

The business world is rife with stories of unequal and condescending treatment of women in the C-suite. Until the last few decades, inappropriate comments and outright sexual harassment were routine and received little or no attention; more recently, such issues have become the focus of heightened scrutiny and new workplace guidelines and regulations. Still, many improper behaviors continue. An organization that hopes to be an employer of choice for female leaders must take a proactive approach to eliminating any semblances of harassment. The following areas of focus can assist in this regard:

- *Avoid stereotypes.* Executives, both male and female, should be aware of gender biases and seek to dispel them at all times. For example, if an organization needs a project manager to evaluate a proposal for a new childcare center, it should not select a female purely because of societal expectations that a woman might be "more caring." The decision should be based on competence.

- *Be mindful of office décor and decorum.* Though office decorations can be a reflection of an individual's personality, standards must be set to prohibit decorations that might be considered sexually suggestive or otherwise offensive to others in the office. Likewise, inappropriate "water cooler" talk or jokes of a sexual nature have no place in a professional environment and should not be tolerated under any circumstances.

- *Follow a strict "hands-off" rule.* Executives should remember that any form of touching other than a handshake might be misinterpreted. Moreover, no communication, whether verbal or nonverbal, should be tolerated if it might be construed in a sexual nature or lead a female peer or subordinate to feel intimidated. The workplace might be a convenient place to meet interesting people, but romantic relationships in the office, even if they are consensual and outside direct reporting lines, often end poorly and decrease the effectiveness of all involved. Leaders should look elsewhere to find a date.

Ensure Pay and Advancement Equity

Even when controlling for level of education and years of experience, research shows that men in executive positions in healthcare continue to earn significantly higher salaries than women in similar positions (ACHE 2012). Pay inequality exacerbates the challenges faced by women leaders, who often are presented with difficult choices between raising a family and advancing in their careers. Leadership teams must be diligent to ensure that similarly qualified executives receive parity in compensation regardless of gender. Leaders also must ensure that historical biases—such as not promoting a young female executive out of fears that she might have children and take time away from the office—are overcome.

Support Balance Between Work and Family Commitments

Female executives commonly face competing demands from their personal and professional lives. For instance, numerous studies have indicated that women typically serve as the primary caregivers of children, especially when the children are sick. Furthermore, women who have children likely face career interruptions of three months or more during the maternity process. Organizations must be aware of these demands and flexible enough to allow women leaders an appropriate work–life balance.

Many women feel they are forced to choose between climbing the organizational hierarchy and having a family, and this perception has likely contributed to the fact that female executives are significantly less likely than their male counterparts to aspire to CEO positions (ACHE 2012). Such lowered aspirations represent a tremendous lost opportunity for healthcare organizations. Talented women leaders should be shown that they have a wider array of options and that they can raise a family without sacrificing their career advancement. Many organizations offer hybrid programs that allow new mothers to ease back into their professional roles by working remotely from home; such arrangements can help minimize concerns of having to rush back to the office to avoid losing traction on the corporate ladder. Affording female executives the opportunity to attend important events in the lives of their children, to take vacations during school holidays, and to use affordable childcare alternatives (including sick child care) can all help attract talented female leaders to an organization.

SUMMARY

The demography of the United States is undergoing a tremendous evolution. With birth rates declining among Caucasians and holding steady among African Americans and Hispanics, groups that historically have been considered minorities will soon make up a majority of the population. This shift is changing the face of the workforce and patient population for nearly every healthcare delivery system in the country. To appropriately serve these evolving constituencies, healthcare leaders must fundamentally embrace the concept of diversity in their organizations, and they must develop the competencies necessary to foster a culture of inclusivity. Only through the concerted efforts of leaders at all levels will the gaps in ethnic and gender equality be closed and the most effective approaches to healthcare management be achieved.

GUEST COMMENTARY: KELVIN A. BAGGETT

Inclusiveness is a word that is frequently used but not as frequently practiced. To me, it means not just having someone seated at the decision-making table but also inviting and encouraging that individual to participate in the decision. This view supports the findings that continue to emerge on having the wisdom of a team shape decisions and leveraging different perspectives to offer views that might not otherwise be considered.

As a leader, I find it most fulfilling to have diversity on my team. That diversity is not limited to race and ethnicity, which most frequently come to mind, but also includes such aspects as gender and professional background. My goal, however, is not to merely have these diverse individuals listed as members of the team, but to have them as welcome voices and contributors. To help everyone understand the importance of having diversity represented and heard, my organization has an operating principle and an operating model.

Our operating principle is that we seek the most qualified applicant for each position. The process for selection involves asking a simple question, "What out-of-the-box approach or talent can help us to solve the problem that we have outlined or capture the opportunity that we have identified?" This simple thought process helps us think beyond a traditional replacement approach and consider alternative candidates for the role. With our principle, we are not only embracing and promoting our philosophy to think differently; we are also pushing ourselves to challenge one another in the selection process. Ultimately, we are seeking the best fit and feel.

(continued)

(continued from previous page)

Our operating model promotes a culture in which the leadership team has an obligation to dissent. Instead of seeking to suppress challenges and debates, we actively seek to promote them in a respectful and dignified fashion. We believe that raising questions and challenging one another help us to shape a better approach and gain the necessary ownership for implementation and sustainability.

Kelvin A. Baggett, MD
Senior Vice President, Clinical Operations,
and Chief Clinical Officer
Tenet Healthcare Corporation
Dallas, Texas

REFLECTIVE QUESTIONS

1. Think back to the last search you conducted to fill a leadership vacancy. What did you do in the selection process to promote diversity? How could the concepts outlined in this chapter have enhanced the process?

2. In reviewing the leadership of your own organization, how well does the makeup reflect that of the community you serve? If gaps exist, how might you approach working with your leadership team to raise awareness?

RESOURCES AND EXERCISES FOR LEADERSHIP DEVELOPMENT

1. Review the American College of Healthcare Executives (ACHE) policy statement on diversity, titled "Increasing

and Sustaining Racial/Ethnic Diversity in Healthcare Management" (www.ache.org/policy/minority.cfm).

2. Attend a local or national meeting of the Asian Health Care Leaders Association (www.ahcla.org), the National Association of Health Services Executives (www.nahse.org), the National Forum for Latino Healthcare Executives (www.nflhe.org), or the Rainbow Healthcare Leaders Association (www.rhla.org).

3. Become familiar with the Institute for Diversity (www.diversityconnection.org).

REFERENCES

American College of Healthcare Executives (ACHE). 2015. "CEO Research Findings: 2014 Survey of Career Attainments of Healthcare Executives by Race/Ethnicity." *Chief Executive Officer* newsletter. Accessed September 30. www.ache.org/newclub/newslttr/ceo/CEO-Circle-Newsletter/CEOnewsletter_Summer15.pdf.

————. 2012. *A Comparison of the Career Attainments of Men and Women Healthcare Executives.* Published December. www.ache.org/pubs/research/2012-Gender-Report-FINAL.pdf.

American College of Healthcare Executives (ACHE), Asian Health Care Leaders Association, Institute for Diversity in Health Management, National Association of Health Services Executives, and National Forum for Latino Healthcare Executives. 2008. *A Racial/Ethnic Comparison of Career Attainments in Healthcare Management.* Accessed September 21, 2015. www.ache.org/pubs/research/Report_Tables.pdf.

Burns, C., K. Barton, and S. Kerby. 2012. "The State of Diversity in Today's Workforce: As Our Nation Becomes More Diverse So

Too Does Our Workforce." Center for American Progress. Published July 12. www.americanprogress.org/issues/labor/report/2012/07/12/11938/the-state-of-diversity-in-todays-workforce/.

Funderburg, L. 2013. "The Changing Face of America." *National Geographic*. Published October. http://ngm.national geographic.com/print/2013/10/changing-faces/funderburg-text.

Gin, J. 2013. "Thoughts on Newsroom Diversity." Radio Television Digital News Association. Accessed March 31, 2015. www.rtdna .org/content/diversity_toolkit.

Miller, F. S., and J. H. Katz. 2002. *The Inclusion Breakthrough: Unleashing the Real Power of Diversity*. San Francisco: Berret-Koehler.

Taylor, P. 2014. "The Next America." Pew Research Center. Published April 10. www.pewresearch.org/next-america /#Two-Dramas-in-Slow-Motion.

CHAPTER 16

The Multigenerational Workforce

As the US workforce ages, more generations are working alongside each other. The knowledge, skills, and attributes possessed by today's multigenerational workforce present multiple challenges and opportunities to business leaders. Smart employers realize that one of the keys to growing and succeeding in an increasingly competitive global marketplace is recruiting and managing talent drawn from workers of all ages. Leading, and successfully managing, an inter- generational workforce will become a business imperative that few organizations can ignore.

—Society for Human Resource Management

Guide to Reader

Having multiple generations in the workforce is not a new issue, but in today's environment, it is an issue of heightened importance. People now work much later in life than they did in the past (often into their 70s), and the range of ages in the workplace is wider than ever before. Generational differences in attitudes, behaviors, and expectations are significant, and, in service industries such as healthcare, they can often lead to conflict and discord. Leaders must recognize and understand these divergences and manage them effectively.

Respect Your Elders

A bright young leader was making his way through the formal COO development program of a large investor-owned hospital management company. A newly minted MBA from an Ivy League school, he was determined to become a hospital CEO as soon as possible. Early in his administrative fellowship with the organization, he had used his knowledge of social media to start a grassroots campaign to educate patients about new service lines being introduced at the hospital where he was working. The marketing efforts were extremely successful in driving awareness and volumes at minimal cost, and the success raised the young leader's organizational profile and accelerated his progress through the development program.

The executive in charge of the development program soon placed the young leader in an assistant administrator role in charge of support services (security, plant operations, volunteer services, housekeeping, and food services) at one of the company's smaller hospitals. When the assistant administrator met with his department director team for the first time, he was immediately struck by the tenure of the individuals in the room. Three of his directors were in their late 50s, and the director of plant operations was nearing his seventieth birthday. On the opposite end of the spectrum, the food services director was a contract employee in her early 20s who was extremely motivated to be successful in her first leadership role.

The assistant administrator began to lay out his strategy for the departments and informed the group about his preferred communication style, which relied heavily on

(continued)

(continued from previous page)

electronic media such as text messages and e-mail. He also announced that he would post meeting agendas on a shared website he had created for the group and that any edits to the documents could be accomplished using file-sharing software that the company had recently purchased. He encouraged each director to take an active role in shaping discussions by suggesting new agenda topics. He placed the food services director in charge of maintaining the site for the group, as a developmental opportunity.

The assistant administrator scheduled individual standing meetings with his directors for the discussion of important issues related to each department. With the more tenured directors, he felt compelled to bring up the topic of succession planning, because he did not want to be left with vacancies in key areas when the directors retired. He felt that the individual meetings were going well and that he was building an excellent rapport with his team. He was somewhat surprised by the lack of input from his directors into the meeting agendas, but he attributed the silence to the fact that the team was still getting to know him and becoming accustomed his leadership style.

The company conducted a 360-degree evaluation of the new leader 90 days after his start date, and when the assistant administrator received his summary report, he grew very concerned. Only one of his subordinates—the young food services director—was happy with how he was approaching his work. The rest of his team expressed dissatisfaction with his reliance on electronic media as the main platform for sharing information; most preferred

(continued)

(continued from previous page)

face-to-face interaction and exchange of ideas. Furthermore, several of his direct reports took offense to his discussions of succession planning, because many of them still considered themselves to be "midcareer." Given this feedback, the assistant administrator requested additional training in "generational competence" so that he could more effectively lead his team.

Be mindful: Every generation has unique characteristics that differ from those of the generations that came before. Learning to cultivate the strengths that each generation brings and developing teams that foster intergenerational collaboration can create a powerful competitive advantage.

MULTIPLE GENERATIONS AT WORK

For the first time in the history of American industry, four generations are actively engaged in the workforce at the same time: the silent generation, which includes workers born before 1946; the baby boomers, who were born between 1946 and 1964; generation X, born between 1965 and 1980; and generation Y, or millennials, born between 1981 and 2000. Each of these generations has been molded through a distinct set of experiences, and each presents unique opportunities and challenges to workplace leadership. Moreover, because each generation has its own values and motivating factors, the dynamic between representatives from different generations must be managed to avoid unnecessary conflict. The following is a brief summary of the characteristics of each generation:

- The silent, or greatest, generation makes up a smaller percentage of the workforce each year. Members of this generation were shaped by the experiences of the Great Depression and World War II, and they have a strong sense of honor, duty, and loyalty to their organizations. They are not usually motivated by instant gratification or quick financial rewards; rather, they take great pride in their contributions to the overall organizational mission and enjoy being part of something larger than themselves.

- The baby boomers were born to the throngs of soldiers returning from World War II, and the generation developed during a time of prosperity in the United States that extended into the 1950s and early 1960s. Baby boomers' lives were shaped by periods of great turmoil and social change. They lived through the war in Vietnam, the civil rights movement, economic crises in the 1970s and 1980s, and the Wall Street merger and acquisition binges that caused significant job loss. One thing baby boomers inherited from their parents was a strong work ethic. They often measure work ethic by the number of hours worked per week, and they are considered highly loyal to the companies for which they work. The baby boom generation has also been described as the "me" generation, reflecting an emphasis on being financially rewarded in proportion to the efforts expended.

- Members of generation X have been greatly influenced by the strong work ethic of their baby boomer parents. Many generation Xers grew up as "latchkey kids" in households where both parents pursued careers, and they often had little supervision or adult guidance during childhood. As a result, generation X is largely made up of self-starters who do not require or respond well to micromanagement. They generally approach life with a healthy dose of skepticism, and because many generation Xers saw their parents' devotion to a company rewarded with downsizing and job loss, their loyalty typically lies with individuals rather than with firms.

- Generation Y, also known as millennials, is the fastest-growing segment of the workforce, and it now holds a majority of entry-level positions. Many millennials were reared by early generation X parents who vowed to be different from their absentee parents; as a result, young millennials often were smothered with attention and praise and had their days carefully scheduled with various activities. Accordingly, millennials in the workforce are often highly dependent on a structured environment and look for constant direction from supervisors. This generation also graduated from college around the time of the Great Recession, so they have resigned themselves to careers with multiple job changes and a variety of employers.

Leaders should be aware of the risk of relying too heavily on broad generalizations, because the rules all have numerous exceptions. Still, familiarity with key aspects of each generation's behaviors, needs, and career approaches can help promote working relationships built on mutual understanding. Exhibit 16.1 provides a brief reference summary for leaders managing a multigenerational workforce.

MANAGING A MULTIGENERATIONAL WORKFORCE

Because of the generations' differing skills, motivations, and desires, leaders must adapt their individual management styles to create an environment that maximizes the strengths of all workers and leverages the unique perspectives that the workers bring to a team. When managers view generational differences as strengths, the potential for collaboration is powerful. The following protocol,

EXHIBIT 16.1: Generational Attributes

Generation	Birth Years	Estimated Percentage of Workforce in 2015	Work Perspectives
Silent, or greatest, generation	1922–1945	Approximately 10%	Emphasize company loyalty and strong work ethic
Baby boomers	1946–1964	44%	Live to be in the office; include the first generation of women to enter workforce in large numbers
Generation X	1965–1980	34%	Believe that work should not define their lives, look for work–life balance, loathe micromanagement
Generation Y, or millennials	1981–2000	12%	Desire meaningful work; are socially conscious and technologically savvy

Source: Data from Toossi (2012).

which is summarized in Exhibit 16.2, can assist leaders in managing a multigenerational workforce and helping members of all generations to lead fulfilling professional lives.

EXHIBIT 16.2: Protocol for Managing a Multigenerational Workforce

The following framework can provide guidance to leaders who manage workers from multiple generations:

1. Honor the greatest generation.
2. Leverage the strengths of the boomers.
3. Serve generation X.
4. Mentor the millennials.

Honor the Greatest Generation

The term "greatest generation," coined by Tom Brokaw (1998), references the fact that members of the silent generation endured the struggles of the Great Depression and fought valiantly in World War II. The presence of these individuals in the workforce—even in dwindling numbers—represents a tremendous resource to leaders and staff that will soon be lost. In a healthcare organization, these individuals represent the senior physicians, leaders, and frontline caregivers who have likely been with the organization for many years. Not only do they have tremendous wisdom to bestow on the other generations; they also serve as organizational historians. Many serve as volunteers and come to the facility after a successful career in other industries, reflecting a true desire to help others. Using members of the silent generation as a resource, even for a short time, and leveraging their skills for the mentorship of younger workers can transmit and preserve valuable lessons about work ethic and organizational loyalty.

Leverage the Strengths of the Boomers

The baby boomer generation represents both the greatest asset and the greatest risk in healthcare today. Many baby boomers hold key administrative and clinical leadership roles, and as they reach retirement age, their exodus will represent an enormous loss of stability and knowledge. Furthermore, because the generations that have followed the boomers are smaller in number and typically do not share the same work ethic, attempting to backfill positions as boomers leave the workplace will be extremely difficult. Compounding the challenge for healthcare organizations is the fact that baby boomers will be significant drivers of demand for healthcare services as they reach their golden years. In short, the aging of baby boomers creates both supply and demand challenges for healthcare. Leaders can help slow this out-migration and leverage the strengths of boomers for as long as possible through the following actions:

- *Provide stability.* More than any generation before them, the baby boomers have experienced tremendous volatility in their careers. Leaders should be mindful of this dynamic and offer programs to provide boomers with a sense of stability as they approach retirement age. Some healthcare facilities have even begun to offer "trial retirement" programs that allow boomers to maintain full-time benefits while tapering down their work schedules on a multiyear glide path to retirement.
- *Motivate with financial rewards.* Remember that the baby boomers are known as the "me" generation, and they generally respond well to financial rewards for the value they bring to an organization. Many boomers are looking to pad their "nest egg" for retirement, and financial incentives can be a powerful tool to influence their behavior. Rather than simply linking financial incentives to traditional productivity, some organizations provide bonuses to boomers based on their willingness to mentor entry-level staff and midlevel leaders and to help bridge generation gaps.

Serve Generation X

While overachieving baby boomers put in long hours at work, their children—members of generation X—often spent much of their youths with babysitters, television, and video games. The relative lack of parental guidance created a generation of self-starters who can succeed with little direction, but it also led generation Xers to place a greater emphasis on work–life balance than the workers who preceded them. Less receptive to the traditional top-down hierarchical management style of the past, generation X responds well to inclusive leadership and enjoys being involved in the decisions that affect their work. Essentially, they respond better to broad guidance than to micromanagement. Generation X is critically important right now because its members occupy a majority of middle-management roles and will soon take over senior leadership. To maximize the satisfaction and output of generation Xers, consider the following tactics:

- *Remember that actions speak louder than words.* Many generation Xers saw their parents put in long hours at the office only to be laid off because of downsizing or outsourcing. As a result, they are often skeptical of organizational leadership and judge leaders by their actions rather than by their words. Promises of fast-track promotional opportunities will not impress members of this generation; they are looking for what you can provide to them today.
- *Do not micromanage.* Members of generation X respond best to broad guidance and feedback. Having been raised in largely unstructured environments, many are turned off by overly prescriptive management styles.
- *Provide flexibility and balance.* Though generation Xers demonstrate a strong work ethic, they are focused more on output and results than on the number of hours worked. They are not opposed to working occasional evenings or weekends to achieve results, as long as they are able to attend such events as a child's after-school play or soccer game. Because generation X values work–life balance, organizations can improve motivation and retention of these employees by allowing them the flexibility to manage their own schedules (within reason) as long as results are achieved.

- *Praise frequently.* Having grown up largely as latchkey kids, many generation X workers crave feedback on their job performance. Providing frequent and informal praise can boost productivity and align the behavior of this generation with the organization's goals.

Mentor the Millennials

Millennials grew up in the most structured environment of any generation to date, the result of so-called "helicopter parents" who hovered over them and planned every aspect of their lives. Generation Y workers therefore tend to thrive in a structured work environment and rely heavily on the direction of supervisors. Because such tendencies are diametrically opposed to those of generation X, conflicts between the two generations are common and require careful management. Both generations X and Y work well in teams, so assigning a millennial to a team with a generation X mentor can help bridge this gap. Generation Y is an especially values-driven and technologically savvy generation, and it has great strengths to contribute to the workplace if managed appropriately. The following tactics can assist in this regard:

- *Provide meaningful work.* Millennials have come to expect that their careers will involve multiple employers and, as technology advances, perhaps multiple fields. To that end, this generation is highly motivated by roles that will allow them to build their skill sets and improve their future career prospects; such considerations likely matter more than pay or title.
- *Encourage appropriate use of technology.* Millennials were raised on technology and often feel more comfortable texting than they do having a face-to-face conversation. Rather than discourage their habits, set appropriate

ground rules for their use of technology and leverage their knowledge in projects that have a technology component. Also, because generation Y is accustomed to instant gratification, texting a quick note of praise or thanks will likely resonate well.

- *Provide guidance.* Many millennials grew up with every aspect of their lives managed for them, so helping them transition to the workforce as independent professionals can be tricky. Pairing them with a strong mentor or preceptor can greatly enhance the likelihood of success and retention. Engaging millennials' parents in discussions about a job and benefits can also be helpful. In fact, many hospitals now request that millennials bring a parent to a meeting after a job offer has been extended, to promote better understanding of the benefits structure and expectations of the role.

SUMMARY

At no other time in our history has there been such diversity of ages in the workforce. As members of different groups bring their unique lenses and experiences to organizations, leaders face the challenge of adapting their management styles to maximize the strengths of the various constituencies and ensure effective inter-actions. To be successful, organizations must address a variety of issues related to this multigenerational environment. Moreover, they must adjust their cultural norms to emphasize the respect for and value of all workers and truly appreciate those workers' differences.

GUEST COMMENTARY: GERRY IBAY

I am honored to offer a guest commentary for this chapter on multigenerational workforce dynamics. I agree with Carson and Brett that "[i]n healthcare, leadership is, at its core, a business of building and maintaining positive relationships." Creating and sustaining positive relationships is tricky enough on its own; it's even trickier when it has to be done across multiple generations. Carson and Brett highlight some very important considerations in addressing multiple generations to build such relationships.

I'm a generation Xer, and I definitely value autonomy—sometimes to a fault. I want to add value to my organization and deliver on specific outcomes, but with a great deal of flexibility on my choice of and adherence to processes. Like many gen Xers, I believe I work most creatively and effectively when allowed a certain level of independence. But sometimes I fail to recognize when I'm in over my head (or I know I'm in too deep but am too afraid to mention anything), and my autonomy quickly tailspins into maverick behavior. So the best way people can work with me and other gen Xers and help us grow in our effectiveness is to allow flexibility within boundaries.

Jesse Carmichael, keyboardist from the band Maroon 5, spoke eloquently about this dynamic. "Structure is like the sides of the river," he said. "In order for the river to flow, you have to have these sides. Otherwise, the river would just spread out and evaporate. Whenever you introduce structure, your energy can flow."

(continued)

(continued from previous page)

Like a river, I can allow my need for freedom to spread me too thin. When this happens, my efforts evaporate into the air, producing no discernible results. I will always want the freedom to run freely, so I often have to discipline myself and provide my own structure. If I need help with the structuring part, people from other generations are often best suited to provide it. By working together across generational lines, we can all benefit from the positive flow of directed energy.

Gerry Ibay
Manager, Clinical Information Systems
New York Presbyterian Hospital
New York, New York

REFLECTIVE QUESTIONS

1. Given their respective backgrounds and work perspectives, why would one expect conflicts between employees from generation X and generation Y? How can they be avoided?

2. What are some ways that you might leverage the strengths of older generations, such as the baby boomers, to help recruit and retain younger workers?

RESOURCES AND EXERCISES FOR LEADERSHIP DEVELOPMENT

1. Meet with a person from a different generation and explore generational differences in detail. If possible, choose someone from a different work area, and not someone

with whom you have a boss–subordinate relationship. The ages should be far enough apart to allow for substantially different viewpoints. For example, a 60-year-old might meet with a 30-year-old. The dialogue need not be scripted, but you may wish to share a chart or article on generational differences and ask whether the person agrees or disagrees. Sources for such charts and articles include the following:

Hammill, G. 2005. "Mixing and Matching Four Generations of Employees." *FDU Magazine Online.* Accessed April 12, 2015. www.fdu.edu/newspubs /magazine/05ws/generations.htm.

LaManna, L. 2012. "An Inside Look at How Gen Y, Gen X and Baby Boomers View the Workplace." *Digitalist.* Published November 14. http://blogs.sap.com /innovation/human-resources/an-inside-look-at -how-gen-y-gen-x-and-baby-boomers-view-the -workplace-020721.

LifeCourse Associates. 2015. "Why Generations Matter." Accessed April 12. www.lifecourse.com/services /generations-in-the-workforce/white-paper/.

2. The *Wall Street Journal* provides an excellent short guide to working with various generations (http:// guides.wsj.com/management/managing-your-people /how-to-manage-different-generations/).

3. Review the following articles:

Dhawan, E. 2012. "Gen-Y Workforce and Workplace Are Out of Sync." *Forbes.* Published January 23. www.forbes.com/sites/85broads/2012/01/23 /gen-y-workforce-and-workplace-are-out-of-sync/.

Ruch, W. 2005. "Full Engagement." *Leadership Excellence* 22 (12): 11.

REFERENCES

Brokaw, T. 1998. *The Greatest Generation*. New York: Random House.

Toossi, M. 2012. "Labor Force Projections to 2020: A More Slowly Growing Workforce." US Bureau of Labor Statistics. Published January. www.bls.gov/opub/mlr/2012/01/art3full.pdf.

PART IV

Capstone

CHAPTER 17

Self-Awareness and Derailment

Becoming self-aware is learning about you and teaching yourself.
As a leader develops self-awareness, he is also developing "others
awareness," and this will lead to better methods of leading and
working in the future.

—LTC John M. Shay, United States Army

Guide to Reader

How would you rate your self-awareness? Do you ever feel
that you are in danger of losing your leadership stride?
The authors believe that self-awareness is the foundation
stone for addressing all the issues presented in this book.
Self-awareness is one of the fundamentals of emotional
intelligence. Simply put, it helps us understand both
ourselves and the ways others perceive us. Self-awareness
is the starting point for all leadership growth, and a lack of
it makes leaders more prone to failure. This chapter serves
as the "capstone" to the book and presents critical insight
into some of the most important realities of leadership.

The Best Advice

At the end of her long, distinguished career in healthcare leadership, Mary was asked to serve as an executive in residence at a well-known health administration program. The following comments are from her opening class to second-year students:

"Let me give you the best advice I can give. Class, this is probably the only time when I think you should take detailed notes on my presentations. First and foremost, our field is special—we are here for those who are weak and need care. Secondly, don't believe in your own press clippings—you are not bigger than the world. Finally, if you don't develop and maintain strong self-awareness throughout your entire career, you very likely will stumble. I have worked 44 years in eight health systems, and I have worked for and with many senior leaders. Here is what got them in trouble: They lost that ability to listen to others. They often thought, because of their experiences, that they had been through it all and that no problem was too big for them to solve. Many of them wanted to win at all costs even if it meant hurting people in the process. Sarcasm and negativity have no place in leadership. Neither does emotional volatility. Do you seem to be a polarizing force in your work setting? If so, figure out why and work to curb it. Don't take credit for something your team did for you. And in meetings, you do not always have to talk; resist your urge to add your own comments when they might simply be repetitive of what has already been said. Be on time and be respectful. Don't play favorites. Admit when you are wrong, and don't try to turn the spotlight on yourself when you're right. And don't ever say, 'I told you so.'"

(continued)

(continued from previous page)

She concluded her speech: "Class, there are many more admonitions and counsel than just these. Seek them out and claim them as your own. It is not all about profitability or market share or being the biggest or the best known. It is about listening to others as they tell you about yourself and addressing your needs to improve."

Be mindful: The extent of our self-awareness will likely correlate positively with our successes, and a lack of self-awareness will almost certainly guarantee derailment.

TWO ESSENTIAL CONCEPTS

All of us are very *human*. As such, we will make mistakes, we will have weaknesses, and we will have opportunities to improve. This capstone chapter focuses on two essential concepts that serve as "bookends" for all the material covered in this book. The first focuses on self-awareness and the critical role it plays in leaders' growth and development. The second explores the well-researched area of managerial derailment—a situation that occurs when humans become a little too *human*. In some respects, this chapter might be the most important in the book: Leaders young and old, seasoned and unseasoned, should pay close attention to these important concepts.

Self-awareness is the ability to see ourselves as others see us, and it is a great leadership strength. Derailment might be considered the flip side of the same coin. First described as "managerial derailment" (Bentz 1985; Lombardo, Ruderman, and McCauley 1988; McCall and Lombardo 1983) and later as "leadership derailment" (McCartney and Campbell 2006), *derailment* simply refers to situations where leaders fail. Usually these failures come after periods

> ### The Cost of Bad Managers
>
> "Bad managers are a major health hazard; they impose enormous medical costs on society, and degrade the quality of life of many people."
>
> *Source:* Hogan, Hogan, and Kaiser (2010).

of success, but derailment can happen to leaders early in their careers as well. A deep understanding of how, why, and when leaders fail will help you avoid similar situations in your own career.

SELF-AWARENESS

If there is a single underlying theme in this book, it is the importance of self-awareness in leadership success. In his comprehensive review of leadership derailment, Inyang (2013, 83) writes that self-awareness is "the very first step in making the needed changes that can help prevent a leader from derailing." Self-awareness can also serve to ward off problem areas in the first place. Self-awareness has multiple components, which are presented in Exhibit 17.1 and described—with corresponding lessons—in the paragraphs that follow.

The first, and perhaps most important, component of self-awareness is introspection—the process of looking within oneself and probing one's state of mind, emotions, and spiritual thoughts. Because it requires time and time alone, introspection is at risk of becoming a lost art given the rapidity of society today. Many readers who have worked in Catholic healthcare organizations likely know the value of religious retreats built around quiet thought and reflection. *The lesson: Take needed time—frequently—to reflect, ponder, and think.*

EXHIBIT 17.1: Components of Self-Awareness
- Introspection
- Self-knowledge—the what and the why
- Feedback
- Feedback analysis
  - Consistency of what we find out and know
  - Reliability of what we find out and know
- Ability to frame self-awareness in descriptors
- Clear understanding of the impact of behavior on others (reflect and assess outcomes)
- Admission that there is a problem
- Comfort living a life of dichotomy

The next component, self-knowledge, takes the next step past introspection. Introspection is the start; self-knowledge is the destination. Self-knowledge includes (a) what we *factually* know about ourselves, (b) how we *feel* about those facts, and (c) what we *do* about those facts. It requires a certain level of wisdom, maturity, and judgment. For the purposes of our analysis, it comprises the "what," the "how," and the "actions" of behavior. It addresses such concepts as self-esteem, self-concept, personal values, attitudes, moods, and personal and professional goals. *The lesson: Consider objectively the what and the how of your behaviors and actions.*

Introspection and self-knowledge are fueled by feedback and by what Drucker (2001) called "feedback analysis." Successful leaders work vigorously to get all types of feedback. They rely on feedback not only in such areas as quality, finances, staff, physicians, and patient satisfaction but also on their personal leadership styles and outcomes. Highly effective leaders also know that, for feedback to be valid, it must be both consistent and reliable. Leaders cannot fall into the trap of listening to yes-people. Nor can they rely repeatedly on the same few people to give them input. Leaders must listen to feedback from multiple sources, including sources that might be negative or critical. *The lesson: Feedback must be received continuously and obtained in a reliable manner to ensure that it is not biased.*

The next component is the ability to accurately frame feedback in objective descriptors. The saying "call it like it is" might be the best label for this component. Consider these comments from a CEO: "I was told that I was not communicating very effectively, but no one would tell me exactly what was harming my effectiveness. It was not until I got my administrative assistant to talk to some of these individuals that I was given concrete examples. After taking this to heart, I was better able to improve my communications." Leaders should strive to remove ambiguity and communicate completely, specifically, and precisely. *The lesson: Feedback must be described accurately and objectively.*

Another important component is the ability to understand clearly the impact our behavior has on others. This understanding requires that we take the feedback we have received, continue to reflect on it, and assess the related outcomes. It fundamentally means that we have an acute awareness of others. Zenger (2014) writes: "[T]he most important element of self-awareness, especially for those who lead organizations, is a clear understanding of the impact they are having on the people around them." *The lesson: As leaders, we affect many lives with our behavior. The best leaders hold this principle in respect and reverence.*

One challenging component of self-awareness is the recognition that some of the behavior you practice causes problems. Campbell, Whitehead, and Finkelstein (2009, 60) write: "The daunting reality is that enormously important decisions made by intelligent, responsible people with the best information and intentions are sometimes hopelessly flawed." And, of course, leaders often have difficulty admitting when they have made wrong decisions. *The lesson: Leaders will make mistakes. Admit them, ask for forgiveness, correct the situation the best you can, and move on.*

A final component of self-awareness is the ability to comprehend dichotomies of behavior. For example, leaders must be bold and "in charge" and yet still humble and able to listen quietly. They need to be strategic, with a far-reaching vision for the organization, yet they must also be tactical in their hour-by-hour and day-by-day decisions. They must be prepared to be autocratic in some interactions and participatory in others. If behavioral contradictions cause internal dissonance, the best solution is frequent reflection leading to strong self-awareness. *The lesson: Do not try to develop one "primary style" of leadership; learn multiple approaches and become ambidextrous.*

Learning from Weaknesses

Popular literature—notably that of Buckingham and Clifton (2001)—suggests that leaders grow best by focusing on their strengths and paying little attention to their weaknesses. We are well aware but highly skeptical of this trend. Instead, we tend to side with Kaplan and Kaiser (2013), who write: "We've seen virtually every strength taken too far: confidence to the point of hubris, and humility to the point of diminishing oneself. We've seen vision drift into aimless dreaming, and focus narrow down to tunnel vision. Show us a strength and we'll give you an example where its overuse has compromised performance and probably even derailed a career." Many significant psychologists joined together in Kaiser's (2009) *The Perils of Accentuating the Positive* to strongly discourage the strengths-only focus in leadership development.

Why the great emphasis on this topic? Through both anecdotal evidence and our long personal histories in leadership development, we have come to believe that leaders develop most by understanding their weaknesses, flaws, and shortcomings and taking action to correct them. With close self-examination and continuing self-awareness, leaders can identify weaker areas in their leadership competencies, work through specific behavioral issues, and greatly improve their performance. Certainly, recognition and understanding of one's strengths can help a leader make positive changes; however, one must be aware that these same strengths can become weaknesses. In their leadership competency model, Dye and Garman (2015) describe a number of ways in which too much strength in a single competency can be detrimental. Consider the supposition that boldness and strong extroversion are indicators of successful leaders: Take these strengths to an extreme, and leaders will become overly confident and take risks that are not warranted. Hogan, Raskin, and Fazzini (1990) and Burke (2006) also have illustrated how strengths can have a "dark side." The belief that leaders can grow solely by focusing on their strengths is illogical.

Reality suggests that weaknesses and blind spots will cause stumbling blocks for all leaders. Self-awareness is the best protection against these risks, and it is a true "friend" of leadership. We like the definition of *self-awareness* offered by van Warmerdam (2015): "Self Awareness is having a clear perception of your personality, including strengths, weaknesses, thoughts, beliefs, motivation, and emotions. Self Awareness allows you to understand other people, how they perceive you, your attitude and your responses to them in the moment." Tjan (2012) writes: "It is self-awareness that allows the best business-builders to walk the tightrope of leadership: projecting conviction while simultaneously remaining humble enough to be open to new ideas and opposing opinions."

Challenges in Self-Awareness

The development of self-awareness is a challenge for many leaders. In some cases, self-awareness might be an early career strength that weakens as leaders move up the ladder. Indeed, more senior leaders tend to be less self-aware. The following are several factors that make self-awareness difficult:

- *Aversion to feedback.* Some leaders simply do not receive feedback. Such a dynamic may exist because of (a) organizational cultures that do not support or encourage feedback; (b) leaders who intimidate others from providing feedback; (c) workplaces in which many leaders are only told "good news"; or (d) leaders who are simply too arrogant and pompous to accept feedback. Some organizations emphasize financial metrics or other quantitative measures but make discussions of interpersonal issues off limits. Less-than-positive feedback might be unpleasant to hear, but it can often be career saving.

- *Reliance on the same feedback sources.* Many leaders feel they gather the necessary feedback through rounding and regular interactions with others. The flaw in this approach is that the feedback comes from the *same* individuals who do the most talking. Leaders would do well to review the concepts of statistical sampling when determining whether the feedback they receive really represents the unvarnished truth.

- *Use of feedback only from direct reports.* The act of going around one's managers or direct reports to hear directly from people who work with those individuals can be a sensitive issue, but it occasionally provides feedback that is more meaningful and granular. Direct reports will sometimes soft-coat issues or summarize them in a manner that underestimates potential concerns.

- *Low self-awareness feeding even lower self-awareness.* Individuals who have low self-awareness often fall into a downward spiral in which they no longer hear feedback that might enhance their self-awareness.

- *Organizational measures of success.* Organizations primarily evaluate leaders on organizational parameters, not personal ones. Essentially, leadership success focuses almost entirely on organizational results and not on how those results are attained.

- *Inability to walk in another's shoes.* Lipman (2014) asks the question, "How would you experience your actions if you were on the receiving end?" The most effective leaders are the ones who can see themselves as others see them. As one CEO remarked, good leaders "do not believe so much in their press clippings that they lose sight of their roots and what made them what they are."

- *Mental chatter.* Mental chatter, or noise, is the "conversation" that goes on constantly in our minds. It is not "hearing voices" so much as carrying on internal discussions and deliberations that clog our thoughts. Though mental chatter is a natural part of who we are, it can curb our ability to listen, pay attention, and understand what others tell us. Sometimes mental chatter is like background white noise; other times, it is a more active and assertive voice. In either form, mental chatter can greatly restrict our self-awareness.

Methods to Enhance Self-Awareness

A leader's self-awareness can be enhanced through a variety of methods, activities, and tools. Some approaches can be taken individually, whereas others are taken organizationally. Individual methods for improving self-awareness include the following:

- *Begin with an open mind.* Kurland (2000) relates self-awareness directly to critical thinking and states that critical thinkers "do not take an egotistical view of the world" but instead "are open to new ideas and perspectives." Successful leaders show a sincere and hungry curiosity toward others, and this curiosity, in turn, enhances self-awareness. Consider this: Leaders who can regulate their emotional and judgmental viewpoints are better attuned to others' feelings, beliefs, and emotions. The more open leaders are to others, the more creative their teams are.
- *View self-awareness strategically.* Highly effective leaders view self-awareness as a long-term strategic benefit, and

they understand the power of emotion in self-awareness and in interactions with others. Hogan and Benson (2008) argue that "strategic self-awareness" requires being aware of our internal thoughts and emotions while also having an external view of ourselves. Distinguishing strategic self-awareness from more traditional views of self-knowledge, they write: "The mainstream (and dominant) intrapsychic tradition of personality psychology defines self-knowledge in terms of becoming aware of thoughts and emotions (and strengths) that were formerly unconscious. This is sometimes popularly expressed as getting in touch with one's emotions, strengths (or even one's 'inner child'). This definition of self-awareness is the cornerstone of traditional psychotherapy, and it would be difficult to overstate how influential it has been. In our view, it is also incorrect, and it takes the process of guided individual development in the wrong direction. . . . [S]trategic self-awareness cannot be gained in vacuo or through introspection. Strategic self-awareness depends on performance-based feedback using some sort of systematic assessment process" (Hogan and Benson 2008).

- *Practice active listening.* Active listening requires full attention to the speaker, good eye contact, appropriate body language, and the elimination of distractions (such as e-mail notifications or other interactions with one's computer or smartphone). Perhaps most important, active listening involves trying to discern the reason behind the message as much as the message itself.

- *Learn three old tricks of listening.* Effective leaders have long relied on three "tricks" in situations where close listening and thorough comprehension are especially important (see Exhibit 17.2). The first trick is simple: Repeat back to the communicator what she said to you. Sometimes called "mirroring," this technique ensures that you have

EXHIBIT 17.2: Three Tricks of Effective Listening
1. Repeat back what you have heard (mirroring).
2. Ask questions to amplify and clarify meaning.
3. Summarize. Conclude by listing what was said.

heard correctly what was said. The second trick is to use questions to amplify and clarify the message. Questions demonstrate respect to the speaker and encourage her to provide more depth, texture, and details. The final trick involves summarizing what was said and what was decided during a conversation.

- *Develop a personal SWOT analysis.* Analysis of strengths, weaknesses, opportunities, and threats (SWOT) is a tool widely used in strategic planning, and it can be similarly helpful in enhancing one's self-awareness. Leaders who are highly self-aware know their strengths, their weaknesses, their opportunities for growth and improvement, and the threats that their weaknesses can cause. Moreover, they are comfortable asking for help. Many highly successful leaders use executive or leadership coaching regularly.

- *Keep focus and keep at it.* Developing self-awareness is not something that is done once a year or on the rare occasion that a leader has some downtime. Instead, highly effective leaders regularly carve out time for reflection and engagement inside their minds. Moreover, they are able to hold this focus for long periods. Often, proper reflection requires leaving the smartphone in another room, turning off the cute "whistle" sound for incoming e-mails, or even leaving the office to find a quiet place. See Exhibit 17.3 for some words of wisdom.

EXHIBIT 17.3: Wisdom from Others on Introspection

- "Look for patterns in events you have experienced, behaviors you have engaged in, attitudes that you hold" (Lee and King 2000, 58).
- "Everything that irritates us about others can lead us to an understanding of ourselves" (Jung 1965, 247).
- "Discovering your True North takes a lifetime of commitment and learning. Each day, as you are tested in the real world, you yearn to look in the mirror and respect the person you see and the life you lead" (George 2007).
- "Arrogance, from an organizational leadership perspective, is a kind of blinding belief in your own opinions. . . . Unfortunately, most leaders today operate under highly stressful circumstances where they don't see how their actions are hurting themselves and their companies" (Dotlich and Cairo 2003, 2).

Though individual efforts can be extremely effective in enhancing self-awareness, additional organizational approaches can help produce optimal results. Examples include the following:

- *Create a culture of learning from experience.* Leaders learn best from actual experiences. And according to Thomas (2008, 5), the best experiences are "crucible" experiences— those "trials or tests that corner individuals and force them to answer questions about who they are and what is really important to them." Dye and Sokolov (2013, 162) write that a "crucible experience is one in which an individual is tested, stretched, or challenged by something real." Organizations that recognize this aspect of leadership development tend to foster heightened self-awareness.

- *Incorporate 360-degree assessment programs.* Because they incorporate the views of multiple raters, 360-degree assessments greatly enhance the statistical significance, or "truth," of feedback. Insight from different perspectives and points of view can also enhance one's own self-understanding. To ensure the most useful feedback possible, 360-degree programs must be carefully developed; the guidelines in Exhibit 17.4 can assist in this task.

- *Ensure that the performance management system is viewed positively.* Organizations should have robust performance management systems that leaders appreciate. Rather than approaching performance management as they would a root canal, leaders should value the opportunity for open communication across all areas of performance. Dye and Garman (2015, 192) note: "Leaders who receive higher-quality feedback on an ongoing basis develop faster than those who do not." People benefit most from systems that include (a) well-developed job expectations ("I know what is expected of me"); (b) measurable expectations ("The requirements of my job are quantifiable"); (c) frequent informal feedback ("I hear about how I am doing frequently"); (d) frequent formal feedback ("I hear formally about how I am doing"); and (e) training and development opportunities ("I am given the training and explanations I need to do my job effectively"). Interestingly, the higher up in an organization people move, the less robust the performance management system becomes.

- *Build self-awareness tools and assessments into ongoing leadership development.* The Myers-Briggs Type Indicator and the three well-known Hogan Assessments (the Hogan Personality Inventory; the Hogan Development Survey; and the Motives, Values, and Preferences Inventory) are excellent tools for enhancing self-awareness.

- *Provide executive and leadership coaching.* Many organizations arrange for external parties to serve as coaches to their leaders. Coaching that reflects both expertise and outside objectivity can provide great benefits to leaders at all levels.

EXHIBIT 17.4: Guidelines for Effective 360-Degree Assessment Programs
- Design the questions carefully, and avoid ambiguous terms.
- Keep the survey short and simple.
- Focus on both strengths and weaknesses.
- Ensure that the responses are received and managed by a neutral and trusted third party who has experience with this type of data.
- Ensure that no comments can be traced to individuals.
- Ensure an adequate number of participants (at least six, generally).
- Be clear about the use of the survey data.
- Provide space for qualitative comments.

DERAILMENT

Now let's turn the coin from self-awareness to derailment. As defined earlier, derailment is simply the process whereby leaders fail. Much research on the topic is based on the idea that derailment occurs when a high-potential manager who was expected to advance in an organization fails to do so (Lombardo and McCaulcy 1988). Some literature applies the term *derailment* more specifically to failure that occurs after a period of success, or to more seasoned leaders. For the purposes of our review, however, the lessons of derailment are pertinent to leaders of any age or experience level.

Derailment comes at a great expense to organizations, but the human costs—including job loss, financial hardship, family difficulties, and loss of self-esteem—can be even worse. And despite extensive research on leadership development, derailment remains all too common. Conlow and Watsabaugh (2013) write: "So much research and so many books have been written on supervision, management, and leadership, and yet research shows that 50 percent to 60 percent of managers fail." Wan (2011) reports similar findings: "Although considerable efforts have been spent on leadership development research exploring the reasons for success in managerial or executive roles, about half of all managers nevertheless fail."

> **Derailment Learning Lesson**
>
> Derailment follows recurrent mistakes and problems, most of which produce signs and warnings. Strong self-awareness ensures that alarms go off in time for the leader to act.

Derailment does not occur as the result of a single mistake or misstep; rather, it occurs when leaders have *recurrent* problems with their leadership effectiveness. It involves patterns of behavior that cause errors over time that ultimately lead to job loss. McCall and Lombardo (1983) attribute ultimate derailment to a combination of managerial inadequacies and personal flaws. Hogan, Curphy, and Hogan (1994, 499) suggest that failed leaders have had an "overriding personality defect or character flaw that alienated their subordinates and prevented them from building a team."

Dye and Sokolov (2013, 183) devote an entire chapter of their physician leadership book to the topic of derailment. They observe: "Many physicians who have had a stellar clinical career and positive beginnings in early leadership positions may begin to fall short of what is needed to succeed at the highest levels of the organization." But physicians are not the only profession faced with these problems. All leaders run the risk of derailment.

Common Causes of Derailment

The derailment literature includes numerous studies on the reasons that leaders lose their track. In one of the older studies, Bentz (1985) offered a host of reasons—shown in Exhibit 17.5—that still resonate today. Notice a commonality among the reasons: Many of them emanate from personality and interpersonal issues involved in forming and leading teams. Leadership is not a solo activity, and leaders who try to go it alone risk failure. Popular definitions of both *management* and *leadership* involve "getting things done

EXHIBIT 17.5: Failed Leaders

Failed leaders
(a) lacked business skills,
(b) were unable to deal with complexity,
(c) were reactive and tactical,
(d) were unable to delegate,
(e) were unable to build a team,
(f) were unable to maintain relationships with a network of contacts,
(g) let emotions cloud their judgment,
(h) were slow to learn, and
(i) were seen as having an "overriding personality defect."

Source: Bentz (1985).

through other people." People who are not effective with others will have trouble being successful leaders. One of the earlier theories of leadership aimed to contrast leaders' concern for people with their concern for production; in reality, successful leaders must have equal concern for both.

Leaders must have early-warning systems for any problems that might be surfacing and bringing them closer to derailment. They should carefully monitor their own behavior for such signs as changes in leadership style, often becoming more authoritative and less collaborative; overconfidence; mood changes; interpersonal problems, often caused by the introduction of a new team member; strategic pressures with no clear-cut solutions; and problems in the leader's personal life. Remaining watchful for these common contributors to derailment brings us back full circle to self-awareness—and the need for humility to hear others and to discern one's own effectiveness level.

Correlation Between Derailment and Self-Awareness

We believe that an inverse relationship exists between self-awareness and derailment (see Exhibit 17.6). When self-awareness rises, the chances of derailment decrease; when self-awareness falls, derailment becomes more likely. As leaders grow in experience and seasoning, they tend to rely on the instincts and knowledge they have accumulated over the years. Though knowledge and experience are typically considered strengths, they can quickly turn to weaknesses if a leader grows overconfident, develops an attitude of "I've seen that before," and becomes less likely to seek out or even listen to input from others. A leader's need for awareness and humility was powerfully highlighted in a University of Minnesota study: "[I]nability or unwillingness to see one's own faults is associated with significant career stalling or even derailment. . . . [P]eople who are significant self-promoters—those considered to be out-of-touch with how their direct manager rated them—were 629 percent more likely to derail than the in-touch group" (Quast 2012).

EXHIBIT 17.6: The Inverse Relationship Between Self-Awareness and Derailment

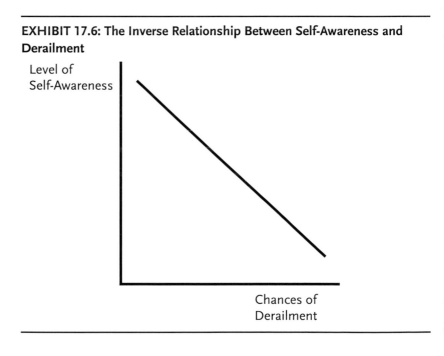

Level of
Self-Awareness

Chances of
Derailment

SUMMARY

Know yourself. Know how others perceive you. Know how your behaviors and actions might harm or curb leadership effectiveness. Practice humility. Shun arrogance and overconfidence.

REFLECTIVE QUESTIONS

1. The chapter's opening questions asked how you would rate your self-awareness and whether you ever feel you are in danger of losing your leadership stride. Are your answers different now that you have read the chapter? How?

2. Take a moment to consider the benefits of a leadership coach. The American College of Healthcare Executives provides an extensive listing of coaches who work primarily in the healthcare field (www.ache.org/newclub/career /execcoach/intro.cfm).

RESOURCES AND EXERCISES FOR LEADERSHIP DEVELOPMENT

1. Review the article "Management Derailment: Personality Assessment and Mitigation" by Hogan, Hogan, and Kaiser (www.veritaslg.com/assets/files/Articles /Coaching/Management%20Derailment.pdf) to gain a more comprehensive understanding of derailment from a psychological perspective.

2. Take some of the sample assessments available online and discuss the results with someone who knows you well. As a general guide, source material from universities' websites— with addresses ending in .edu—tend to be the best. Other useful sources include the following:

- Free Management Books (www.free-management
  -ebooks.com/dldchk/dlchpp-self.htm)
- Bill George (www.billgeorge.org/files/media/true
  -north1/chapter4exercises.pdf)

REFERENCES

Bentz, V. J. 1985. "Research Findings from Personality Assessment of Executives." In *Personality Assessment in Organizations*, edited by H. J. Bernardin and D. A. Bownas, 82–144. New York: Praeger.

Buckingham, M., and D. O. Clifton. 2001. *Now, Discover Your Strengths*. New York: Free Press.

Burke, R. J. 2006. "Why Leaders Fail: Exploring the Dark Side." *International Journal of Manpower* 27 (1): 91–100.

Campbell, A., J. Whitehead, and S. Finkelstein. 2009. "Why Good Leaders Make Bad Decisions." *Harvard Business Review* 87 (2): 60–66.

Conlow, R., and D. Watsabaugh. 2013. "How to Avoid Leadership Derailment." *Bloomberg Business*. Published August 9. www.bloomberg.com/bw/articles/2013-08-09/how-to-avoid -leadership-derailment/.

Dotlich, D. L., and P. C. Cairo. 2003. *Why CEOs Fail: The 11 Behaviors That Can Derail Your Climb to the Top—and How to Manage Them*. San Francisco: Jossey-Bass.

Drucker, P. F. 2001. *Management Challenges for the 21st Century*. New York: Harper Business.

Dye, C. F., and A. N. Garman. 2015. *Exceptional Leadership: 16 Critical Competencies for Healthcare Executives*, 2nd ed. Chicago: Health Administration Press.

Dye, C. F., and J. J. Sokolov. 2013. *Developing Physician Leaders for Successful Clinical Integration*. Chicago: Health Administration Press.

George, B. 2007. "Leadership in the 21st Century." Published March 15. www.billgeorge.org/page/leadership-in-the -21st-century.

Hogan, F., G. J. Curphy, and J. Hogan. 1994. "What We Know About Leadership: Effectiveness and Personality." *American Psychologist* 49 (6): 493–504.

Hogan, J., R. Hogan, and R. B. Kaiser. 2010. "Management Derailment." In *American Psychological Association Handbook of Industrial and Organizational Psychology*, Vol. 3, edited by S. Zedeck, 555–75. Washington, DC: American Psychological Association.

Hogan, R., and M. J. Benson. 2008. "Strategic Self-Awareness." Hogan Assessment Systems. Published May 22. http://info .hoganassessments.com/blog/bid/109303/Strategic -Self-Awareness.

Hogan, R., R. Raskin, and D. Fazzini. 1990. "The Dark Side of Charisma." In *Measures of Leadership*, edited by K. E. Clark and M. B. Clark, 343–54. West Orange, NJ: Leadership Library of America.

Inyang, B. J. 2013. "Exploring the Concept of Leadership Derailment: Defining New Research Agenda." *International Journal of Business and Management* 8 (16): 78–85.

Jung, K. 1965. *Memories, Dreams, Reflections*. New York: Vintage.

Kaiser, R. B. 2009. *The Perils of Accentuating the Positive*. Tulsa, OK: Hogan Press.

Kaplan, R. E., and R. B. Kaiser. 2013. *Fear Your Strengths: What You Are Best At Could Be Your Biggest Problem*. Oakland, CA: Berrett-Koehler.

Kurland, D. J. 2000. "What Is Critical Thinking?" *Critical Reading.* Accessed April 2, 2015. www.criticalreading.com/critical _thinking.htm.

Lee, R. J., and S. N. King. 2000. *Discovering the Leader in You: A Guide to Realizing Your Personal Leadership Potential.* San Francisco: Jossey-Bass.

Lipman, V. 2014. "Why the Best Leaders Are Self-Aware." *Forbes.* Published September 16. www.forbes.com/sites/victorlipman /2014/09/16/why-the-best-leaders-are-self-aware/.

Lombardo, M. M., and C. D. McCauley. 1988. *The Dynamics of Management Derailment.* Technical Report No. 34. Greensboro, NC: Center for Creative Leadership.

Lombardo, M. M., M. N. Ruderman, and C. D. McCauley. 1988. "Explanations of Success and Derailment in Upper-Level Management Positions." *Journal of Business and Psychology* 2 (3): 199–216.

McCall, M. W., Jr., and M. M. Lombardo. 1983. *Off the Track: Why and How Successful Executives Get Derailed.* Greensboro, NC: Center for Creative Leadership.

McCartney, W. W., and C. R. Campbell. 2006. "Leadership, Management, and Derailment: A Model of Individual Success and Failure." *Leadership & Organization Development Journal* 27 (3): 190–202.

Quast, L. N. 2012. "Prevent Top Leader Derailment." *Talent Management.* Published September 27. www.talentmgt.com/articles /prevent-top-leader-derailment.

Thomas, R. J. 2008. *Crucibles of Leadership: How to Learn from Experience to Become a Great Leader.* Boston: Harvard Business School Press.

Tjan, A. K. 2012. "How Leaders Become Self-Aware." *Harvard Business Review*. Published July 19. https://hbr.org/2012/07/how-leaders-become-self-aware/.

van Warmerdam, G. 2015. "Self Awareness." *Pathway to Happiness*. Accessed April 2. www.pathwaytohappiness.com/self-awareness.htm.

Wan, K. E. 2011. "Understanding Managerial Derailment." Civil Service College. Published June. www.cscollege.gov.sg/knowledge/ethos/issue%209%20jun%202011/pages/Understanding-Managerial-Derailment.aspx.

Zenger, J. 2014. "The Singular Secret for a Leader's Success: Self-Awareness." *Forbes*. Published April 17. www.forbes.com/sites/jackzenger/2014/04/17/the-singular-secret-for-a-leaders-success-self-awareness/.

Epilogue

The search for better, more competent leaders, from the presidents of our great companies to our housekeepers, was never more critical than it is now. In times of great change, the need for sound leadership is always in excess of the supply.

—Frederick Winslow Taylor

THE SCIENCE OF LEADERSHIP

Frederick Winslow Taylor (1911), often regarded as the father of modern management theory, wrote the words above in the preface to his seminal work on leadership, *The Principles of Scientific Management*. At the time the book was published, the world was still adjusting to the fundamental social and economic changes of the Industrial Revolution. Taylor felt that the only way the fledgling manufacturing companies could achieve their full human and financial potential was through a top-down hierarchical management structure that governed workers who were judged on how quickly and accurately they performed specific and repetitive tasks.

317

As an engineer for a steel company, Taylor spent countless hours mapping workflow to determine the best ways of performing each operation and the amount of time each operation required. He analyzed materials, tools, and work sequences and established a clear division between management and workers. His base assumption was that the workers of the time, if left to their own devices, would be less likely to work efficiently and improve their productivity. He felt that independent thinking had little, if any, role among the frontline staff.

This theory of "scientific management," as Taylor called it, laid the groundwork for the way most modern organizations are structured, and the concept of task-based division of work still permeates nearly every industry today. More important, Taylor's concepts have formed the basis of leadership preparation—whether in formal education through business schools or in workplace management-training programs—for the past 100 years. The processes of selecting, grooming, and promoting leaders have been largely based on the "hard skills" of management, such as finance and accounting, with success determined, just as it was in the days of Taylor, on the ability to drive efficiency and bottom-line results.

SCIENTIFIC MANAGEMENT EVOLVES

In the years since *The Principles of Scientific Management* was introduced, leaders have found that top-down, task-based leadership can in fact result in role clarity and improved efficiencies. However, they have also found that this approach produces diminishing results in many modern organizations. Today's younger generations generally require more active engagement in decisions that affect their work, and they can quickly become dissatisfied if they feel their leader is not personally vested in their success. In addition, because business strategies are shared widely and evolve quickly in the information age, companies have come to realize that the quality of their people is their only truly sustainable competitive advantage. As a result, organizations can no longer accept the risk of losing talented staff due to abrasive managers. In modern management theory, the manner in which leaders guide their teams to achieve results has become just as important—if not more so—as the actual results that are achieved. In essence, the "soft skills" of leadership have become equally critical to the hard skills.

Contemporary healthcare finds itself in a period of transition not unlike the one faced by the manufacturing industry at the turn of the twentieth century. Societal, demographic, and regulatory changes are causing fundamental shifts in the care delivery model, reimbursement methodologies, and the patient experience. The task-based leadership approach that Taylor promulgated, however, cannot resolve the issues facing today's healthcare leaders. Instead, leaders in healthcare must be able to inspire staff to provide high-quality care and to deliver this care in a customer-friendly manner at efficient price points. This challenge requires that leaders possess skills beyond traditional financial and operational matters; it requires leadership skills for communicating effectively, for building strong teams, for managing relationships with multiple stakeholders, and for not making personal mistakes that damage the culture of the organization. That last point is often the most difficult to learn. It involves the "sense of the appropriate" that highly effective leaders have and that aspiring leaders need to learn.

Whereas the hard skills of financial management, accounting, and operations management can easily be learned in a classroom, the social skills discussed in this book are often learned through trial and error over the course of a career. Unfortunately, some people learn lessons the hard way—through personal and professional failures. The precepts of this book aim to assist leaders in dodging career-ending mistakes and embarrassing business encounters. Clearly, significant skills and motivation will be necessary to navigate the ever-changing waters of our industry.

The French term *faux pas* means *false step*. Our hope for all readers is that your false steps be few and not permanently harmful.

Carson F. Dye
Brett D. Lee

REFERENCE

Taylor, F. W. 1911. *The Principles of Scientific Management.* New York: Harper and Brothers.

Human Resources Ethics Survey

1. Your employment services division quickly reviews applications and resumes and decides which to keep and which to discard based on the initial review. Some of the applications and resumes are placed into a "dead" file, which means that the people to whom they belong will not be considered for any position. This is an acceptable practice.

Strongly agree	Agree	Neither	Disagree	Strongly disagree

2. Discussing family-related issues, such as relocation, with executive candidates is an acceptable practice.

Strongly agree	Agree	Neither	Disagree	Strongly disagree

3. Almost all external applicants deserve an explanation for their rejection when another applicant is selected.

Strongly agree	Agree	Neither	Disagree	Strongly disagree

4. Almost all internal applicants deserve an explanation for their rejection when another applicant is selected.

Strongly agree	Agree	Neither	Disagree	Strongly disagree

5. Aiming to meet diversity goals by designating certain positions to be filled by applicants from minority groups is an acceptable practice.

Strongly agree   Agree   Neither   Disagree   Strongly disagree

6. Employees who are terminated during the probationary period of employment—for example, during the first three months—should have no right to appeal or file a grievance according to organizational procedure.

Strongly agree   Agree   Neither   Disagree   Strongly disagree

7. Certain applicants, such as convicted felons, should never be hired in positions that put them in direct contact with patients.

Strongly agree   Agree   Neither   Disagree   Strongly disagree

8. Unless prohibited by written contract or statute, an employer should have the right to terminate an employee for any cause.

Strongly agree   Agree   Neither   Disagree   Strongly disagree

9. Using hidden surveillance cameras to detect employee theft, especially when such an incident has occurred, is an acceptable practice.

Strongly agree   Agree   Neither   Disagree   Strongly disagree

10. Random locker searches for illegal drugs are acceptable as long as employees are informed beforehand of the possibility.

Strongly agree   Agree   Neither   Disagree   Strongly disagree

11. A competent human resources manager who becomes an active member of a politically extreme group, such as the Ku Klux Klan, should be terminated.

Strongly agree   Agree   Neither   Disagree   Strongly disagree

12. A competent night-shift boiler operator who becomes an active member of a politically extreme group, such as the Ku Klux Klan, should be terminated.

Strongly agree   Agree   Neither   Disagree   Strongly disagree

13. Making personal phone calls at work is an acceptable practice.

Strongly agree   Agree   Neither   Disagree   Strongly disagree

14. After employees surpass ten years of service, an employer has a social responsibility to sustain their employment as long as they are not guilty of serious misconduct on the job. Sustaining may mean retraining for new jobs, reassignment to other areas, or creating work.

Strongly agree   Agree   Neither   Disagree   Strongly disagree

15. When a personality clash exists between an employee and her supervisor and no other jobs exist to which either party can easily be transferred, terminating the employee, not the supervisor, is an acceptable practice.

    Strongly   Agree   Neither   Disagree   Strongly
    agree   disagree

16. Employees should be allowed to use formal grievance procedures only for specific violations of established hospital policies and procedures.

    Strongly   Agree   Neither   Disagree   Strongly
    agree   disagree

17. All employees who steal prescription drugs for any reason should be terminated immediately.

    Strongly   Agree   Neither   Disagree   Strongly
    agree   disagree

18. Certain situations permit a human resources manager to discuss with the boss information that was revealed to him in absolute confidence by an employee.

    Strongly   Agree   Neither   Disagree   Strongly
    agrec   disagree

19. Distorting the truth to protect someone is acceptable practice.

    Strongly   Agree   Neither   Disagree   Strongly
    agree   disagree

20. If the hiring salary range for a particular position is $150,000–$175,000 per year and the top candidate for the position earns only $100,000 per year, then hiring

the person at $125,000 is acceptable practice because no internal equity problems would emerge.

Strongly agree   Agree   Neither   Disagree   Strongly disagree

21. The degree of support for the annual United Way fund drive or another hospital-sponsored charity may be used as a performance criterion in appraising a manager's job performance.

Strongly agree   Agree   Neither   Disagree   Strongly disagree

22. Taking home pencils, paper clips, or other small desk items for personal use is an acceptable practice.

Strongly agree   Agree   Neither   Disagree   Strongly disagree

23. Using the office copier for personal matters, if only for a small number of copies, is an acceptable practice.

Strongly agree   Agree   Neither   Disagree   Strongly disagree

24. Taking a "mental health day" or calling in sick after a busy period at work has ended is an acceptable practice.

Strongly agree   Agree   Neither   Disagree   Strongly disagree

25. People in general give more to an organization than they receive in return.

Strongly agree   Agree   Neither   Disagree   Strongly disagree

SUGGESTIONS

Ethical behavior in human resources situations might be the single greatest determinant of how one's integrity and leadership are perceived by others. The statements in the survey may lack clear-cut answers and often necessitate in-depth assessment to determine a proper course of action. A variety of factors can affect the decisions one makes, but a few key themes are worth noting:

- Many of the statements go straight to the issue of dealing with people fairly. For example, numbers 1, 3, and 4 require leaders to consider how they would wish to be treated. Losing sight of this perspective can cause leaders to choose easy solutions, cut corners, and compromise integrity.
- Some statements, such as numbers 13, 19, 22, 23, and 24, go to the heart of honesty and candor. Often, the practice of "acceptable lying" has compromised the trust that people place in leaders.
- Statements such as those in numbers 2, 5, 6, 8, 9, and 10 illustrate how legal parameters can become comingled with ethical parameters. Not every action that is legal is ethical. Effective leaders use both a knowledge of legalities and an ethical sense of right and wrong.

This survey might be most useful as a management team exercise in which all team members select their answers. Follow-up discussion can then explore the ethical attitudes of fellow team members. Although some of the statements may present questions of legality, the primary intent of this survey is to stimulate discussions along an ethical vein.

Effective Use of LinkedIn

Launched in 2003 as a business-oriented networking website, LinkedIn today has 300 million users in countries throughout the world. As the site continues to grow in prominence, having a well-prepared LinkedIn profile is critical for today's leaders. Regardless of whether you are currently looking for a job, your profile provides a narrative of your career and helps build your brand.

What is the best LinkedIn profile? The answer to this question varies by industry, but a few general guidelines apply to healthcare:

- Have a LinkedIn profile. As simple as it may sound, this step continues to be overlooked by some professionals.
- Provide a personal photo. Keep in mind that this site is focused on you, not your family, your dog, or your favorite vacation destination. A professional photo of yourself in business attire typically works best.
- Carefully consider what e-mail account you will use— work or personal. If you choose a personal account, consider whether you wish for your address to be displayed. Another caveat is that some personal e-mail addresses might convey the wrong impression. For instance, *amazingdriver@mailservice.com* or *bagofchips@ email.com* is likely inappropriate for someone who is adroit in the principles of this book.

- Work diligently to build your number of connections. Ideally, you should aim for 500 plus. At the same time, you should avoid accepting invitations to connect with people with whom you have no true link or connection.
- Carefully design the contents of each section. Your profile is not the place to write a Tolstoy-length novel, nor is it the place to paste in your entire resume. Brief summaries are best. The main sections should be as follows:
  - *Summary.* Be brief, avoid exaggeration, and do not be boring.
  - *Experience.* Here you can list all your career positions. Do not list membership on boards or non-employment-related activities here; there are other locations for those. Again, be brief, and do not try to duplicate an entire resume. Some people suggest listing only basic job functions, whereas others suggest listing major accomplishments—take your choice.
  - *Publications, projects, speaking experience, education, groups.* Here you can list any appropriate non-employment-related activities.

Notes of caution include the following:

- Carefully navigate the sign-up process. If this is your first venture into social media, ask a friend or family member who is adept at these matters for help.
- Manage the privacy settings and be aware of what they mean. Once again, finding that friend or family member can be a great help here. Your privacy settings determine whether your activity will be highly visible or more private.
- Be careful sending out mass invitations to "join your professional network." LinkedIn has a feature that can link to your address book or contacts list and, with a single keystroke, send out hundreds of invitations. These mass

invitations can become a nuisance as they clog people's e-mail in-boxes. Invitations sent in this manner also lose the personal touch and begin to feel more like spam.

- Making changes to your profile can sometimes send the wrong signals to your contacts. For instance, if you change any part of a description or title, your network may see the revision as a job change, even if it is just a wording change. To avoid this problem, learn to "turn off activity updates" when making changes that do not need to be sent to your contacts.

Thanks to Jeremy C. Adams from Cardinal Industries for his help and insight on this section.

Index

Note: Italicized page locators refer to figures or tables in exhibits.

Change: employee engagement and, 99; new CEO and careful path to, 235–36

Character: demonstrating strength of, 33–37; of leader, 54

Checks and balances system: progressive discipline, termination, and, 148

Cheok, L., 243

Chief diversity officers (CDOs), 264

Chief executive officers (CEOs): appointing, governing board and, 128; average tenure for, at hospitals, 206; careful, deliberate path to change and, 235–36; compensation issues and, 11; effective partnering between chief HR officer and, 141, 142; female, 259, 260; high-functioning governing board and, 130, 131; power struggles between board members and, 129; reviewing board functionality and, 136; termination and approval of, 148

Chief human resources officer: changing role of, 142; termination and approval of, 148

Childcare: female executives and, 269

Chinese New Year, 265

Cinco de Mayo, 265

CIOs. *See* Clinically integrated organizations

Civil rights movement, 279

Clarity of communication, 25

Clifton, D. O., 299

Clinically integrated organizations (CIOs), 193

Clinton, Hillary, 259

Cliques, 243

Clothing. *See* Business attire

Coaches: utilizing network of, 52

Coaching: executive or leadership, 304, 306

Code of ethics: organizational, creating and following, 62; professional, adherence to, 63

Code of Ethics (ACHE), 63

Cohn, Kenneth H., 198–99

Collaboration: intergenerational, 278, 280; leader–physician, 184–85, 197, 198–99

Common ground, finding, 115

Communication. *See also* Verbal communication; Written communication: clarity of, 25; digital, 176–77; effective, 19–20, 22, 33; established culture and, 244; importance of, 164–65; leadership and, 161; nonverbal, 251; persuasive, 111; poor, derailment of strategies and, 162–63; professional reputation and, 54; technology and, 172–75, *173*

Community organizations: building professional reputations through, 50

Community programs: diversity and, 265

Compa-ratio, 151–52, *152*

Compensation: race, gender, and, 260; understanding nuances of, 151–52

Competency, 143

Competition: hierarchical management structure and, 106; unhealthy, 108–10

Competitive compensation: perks and, 13

Complaining, avoiding, 98

Complications (Gawande), 60

Compromise, 117

Concise communication, 167–68, *168*

Confidentiality: honoring, recruitment and, 210–11

Confirmation bias, 6, 8

Conflict: healthy, encouraging, 112–13

Conflicts of interest: governing board and, 130; organizational code of ethics and, 62

Conlow, R., 307

Consistency: in executive communication, 171; new role and, guidelines for, 230–31; of personality and management style, 34; self-regulation and, 77

Dye, C. F., 52, 176, 187, 191, 212, 299, 305, 306, 308

Edison, Thomas, 212
Education: advancement of minority groups through, 263
Efficiency, 143
Eichinger, R. W., 6
Eisenhower, Dwight D., 69
Electronic communication: *New York Times* test and, 175
E-mail, 165, 167, 172; being cautious with use of, 116–17; impact of, and confidentiality issues with, 170–71; *New York Times* test and, 175; timely responses to, 174
Emergency Medical Treatment and Active Labor Act (EMTALA), 128
Emotional intelligence, 7; consistency and, 230; empathy, social skills, and, 78–79; enhancing, 74–79; flow of, *74*; protocol for enhancing, *74*; self-awareness and, 75–76, 293; self-regulation and, 77–78
Emotional Intelligence (Goleman), 73
Emotional intelligence quotient (EQ), 74
Empathy, 51, 78–79
Employee development programs: structured, 153
Employees. *See also* Engaging the workforce: benefits cost per, 152, *152*; developing meaningful relationships with, 81; empowering, 93, 99; perception gap between executives and, 7–8; replacing, cost of, 206; retention of, 154; system of due process for, establishing, 145–46
Employment models, 193
EMTALA. *See* Emergency Medical Treatment and Active Labor Act
Engaging the workforce, 87–101; balance, art of leadership, and, 90; developing a staff focus, 91–99, *92*; employee engagement as

leadership mantra, 97; giving up the home field advantage, 95–97; setting a positive tone, 98–99; turning organizational chart upside down, 93–95
Enron accounting scandal, 60
EQ. *See* Emotional intelligence quotient
Ethical behavior: developing deep personal commitment to, 62
Ethical decision making: enhancing, 61–63; modeling, 65
Ethical human resources decisions: making, 146–49
Ethical leadership: protocol for, *61*
Ethics, xx, 143; assessing for specific decisions or actions, 112–13; human resources ethics survey, 321–26; importance of, 60–61
Ethnic discrimination, 260
Ethnic diversity: enhancing, 262–66, *263*
Ethnicity: census data on, 258
Etiquette. *See* Office etiquette
Evans, J. Eric, 38–40
Executive behavior: protocol for, *17*, 17–20
Executive–board partnerships: strong, 133–34
Executive coaching, 304, 306
Executive compensation: leadership perception and, 11–12
"Executive presence": professional image and, 25
Executives. *See also* Chief executive officers: effective communication and, 19; failed, studies on, 21; office culture and actions of, 242; perception gap between front-line staff and, 7–8; perception management as responsibility of, 9–10; replacing, cost of, 206
Executive search firms: reasons for using, *213*; strategic use of, 211–12
Executive suite: as microcosm of organization, 249

Gawande, Atul, 60
Gender, 258; compensation and, 260; pay equity issues and, 268; work–life balance and, 260
Gender diversity: enhancing, *266*, 266–69
Gender equality: 2008 presidential campaign and, 259
Generational differences: viewing as strengths, 280
Generation X, 278; characteristics and attributes of, 279–80; "latchkey kid" childhoods and self-starter abilities of, 279; praise and feedback valued by, 285; work–life balance focus of, 283–84
Generation Y, 278; characteristics and attributes of, 280, *281*; mentoring, 285–86
Gin, J., 258
Goleman, D., 73, 74, 230
Good perceptions: reinforcing and maintaining, 15–16
Governance structure: diverse, assembling, 264
Governing board, 123–38; arming with information, 131–33; building a great board, 130–31; CEO selection and, 128; controversial issues and, 134; effective board relations, 129–36; evolving role of board oversight, 126–29; fiduciary responsibility of, 125, 126, 128; members' community roles, 134; ongoing education for, 132; preference for detail level and, 135; preservation of institutional assets and, 127; quality of care and, 127–28; reviewing functionality of, 136; strong board–executive partnerships, 133–34; time management and, 134; wise management of, 134–36
Graciousness: professional sociability and, 248
Graham, G., 243
Great Depression, 279, 282

"Greatest generation": honoring, 282
Great Recession, 280
Grooming, 37. *See also* Business attire; Professional image; new role and, 227; professional style and, 29
Group practices, 185

Habits: "comfort zones" and, 75
Handshakes, firm, 215
"Hands-off" rule: harassment-free workplace and, 267–68
Handwritten notes, generous use of, 172
Harassment-free workplace: establishing, 267–68
"Hard skills": historic reliance on, 164; of management, 318, 319; MBA degree and, 71
Harvard Business Review, 206
Hawthorne Studies, 250
Hayes, James L., 123
Healthcare: accelerated rate of turnover in, 206; as service and relationship business, 81
Healthcare administration graduate competencies: senior executive's appraisal of, *73*
Healthcare industry: major transition for, navigating, 319
Healthcare leaders: ethical decision making modeled by, 65; perception management and compensation of, 11–12
Healthcare leadership: effective relationships and, 71; importance of ethics in, 61
Healthcare market: competitive compensation and, 151
Healthcare organizations: revamped strategic plans and, 216
Healthcare reform laws: transparency and, 125, 126
Healthcare systems: formal alignment of physicians with, 186
Healthy conflict: encouraging, 112–13
Healthy lifestyle: maintaining, 30–31

Intergenerational collaboration, 278, 280

Internal preparation: effective verbal communication and, 169

Interpersonal relationships: building, new role and, 231; effective leadership and, 69; emotional intelligence and, 74–79; leadership success and, 71, 72, 76; positive, developing and sustaining, 72

Interpersonal skills: "hardwiring" of, 251

Interview panel: running Internet search on, 215

Interview questions: being prepared for, 216; subjective nature of, 207

Interviews: first impressions and, 215; limited reliability of, 206–7; thank-you notes sent after, 215–16

Introspection: self-awareness and, 287, 296; wisdom from others on, 305

Inyang, B. J., 296

Janoso, John "Jack" R., Jr., 234–36

Jargon: avoiding, 171

Jealousy, 108–9

Jennings, Gene, 21

Job analysis: of leadership roles, 208

Job applicants: treating as customers, 209–10

Job loss, 284. See also Termination; Turnover; errors over time and, 308; parents of generation X and, 279

Job specifications: reviewing, 214

Joint Commission, The, 127

Justice: fairness and principles of, 62

Kaiser, R. B., 76, 299

Kant, Immanuel, 139

Kaplan, R. E., 299

Kase, Larina, 25

Katz, J. H., 262

Key facts: knowing and recalling, 20

Knight, P., 6

Kurland, D. J., 302

Labor cost revenue percentage, 146, 147

Laws: HR-related, knowing, 144–46, 156

Lawsuits, 146

Layoffs: ethical human resources decisions and, 146; thoughtful strategy for, 35–36

Layout of office: leadership of organization and, 250

Leaders: balancing internal and external responsibilities of, 44, 50; character of, 54; collaboration between physicians and, 184–85; desired behavior modeled by, 20; effective communication skills and, 175–76; as facilitators, 95; failed, derailment and, 308, 309; human resources roles of, 143; lapses in ethical judgment by, 60–61; objectivity of, characteristics related to, 147; office protocols, core values, and, 249; personal brands defined for, 48; positive tone set by, 98–99; upwardly mobile, "appropriate boldness" and, 107

Leadership: attributes, perceived level of importance in contemporary workplace, 164, 165; balance and art of, 90; communication as lifeblood of, 161; definition of, 176; derailment and, 295; development of, 153; difficult choices, ethical decision making, and, 58–59; diversity in, 259–60, 264; expounding on relationships as basis of, 250–51; learning multiple approaches to, 299; Norman Schwarzkopf on, 36; past, governing board and, 135; physician relationships and stability in, 194; relationship building and, 80–81; relationships as basis of, 71–74; revolving door of, 205–7; roles, formal job analyses of, 208; science of, 317–18; "soft skills" of,

workforce, 250; technology and, 285–86

Miller, F. S., 262

Minority candidates: leadership positions and, 264

Minority–majority population shift: diversity and, 269

Mirroring, 303–4, *304*

Mistakes: admitting to, 115

Modern management theory, 319

Monthly turnover metric, 154

Morality: absolute principles of, 62

Morita, Akito, 203

Motivation, 143

Motives, Values, and Preferences Inventory, 306

Mulcahy, Anne M., 87

Multicultural environment: creating, 263–64

Multiculturalism, 261

Multigenerational workforce, 251, 275–90; generational attributes in, *281*; honoring greatest generation, 282; interpreting appropriate style for, 29; leveraging strengths of baby boomers, 282–83; managing, 275, 280–86, *281*; mentoring the millennials, 285–86; respect your elders, 276–78; serving generation X, 283–85; summary of characteristics in, 278–80

Murdock, T. R., 126

Myers-Briggs Type Indicator, 306

Myspace, 174

Names: remembering, 247

National Association of Health Services Executives, 259

National Forum for Latino Healthcare Executives, 259

National Quality Forum: healthcare trustees survey, 128

Neatness of office, 246

Negative perceptions: effective management of, 14–16

Nepotism: avoiding, governing board and, 131

New role: consistency and, 230–31; looking the part, 226–27; mastering, 226–35; 1-1-3-7 guide and, 231–33; plan for success, 227–28; protocol for success in, *226*; respect and, 235; self-awareness, avoiding derailment, and, 233; structured onboarding plan and, 225; understand, then execute, 229–30

New York Times test: electronic communication and, 175

Nickerson, R. S., 6

Nonverbal communication, 251

Nonverbal messages: awareness of, 168

Not-for-profit providers: state caps on income levels for CEOs of, 11

Obama, Barack, 259

Objective speech, 117

Objectivity: human resources laws and regulations and, 147; of leaders, characteristics related to, *147*

"Occupy Wall Street" movement, 11

Office, The, 239

Office culture: toxic, 242

Office etiquette: appropriate, 242–52; attention to details and, 247; executive, xx, 32; guarding against too much informality, 248–49; keep personal and professional lives separate, 244–45; know and respect the culture, 243–44; professional implications of, 240–41; professional sociability and, 248; protocol for, *243*; view your actions through the eyes of others, 246–47

Office politics, 117–18; accountability and, 113–14; celebrating your successes, 111–12; effective, barriers to, 108–10; effective, protocol for, *111*; healthy conflict and, 112–13; jealousy, 108–9; lesson in, 104–6; navigating through, 243; organizational "rules of engagement" and,

Personal values, 297

Phillips, J. M., 208

PHOs. *See* Physician–hospital organizations

Physician advisory groups, forming, 199

Physician dynamics: changes in, 184–87

Physician–hospital organizations (PHOs), 193

Physician liaison positions: establishing, 190

Physicians: accommodating schedules of, 192; building healthy relationships with, 81, 190–91; as business partners, *186, 193*–95; as clinicians/caregivers, *186,* 187; collaboration between leaders and, 184–85; connecting with, *186;* as customers, *186, 188,* 188–93; derailment of, 308; honoring role of, 189–90; increased engagement between hospitals and, 183, 184–87; involving in strategy, 191; lapses in ethical judgment by, 60; in private practice, shrinkage of, 186; as professional friends, 195–97, *197;* relationships with, 181–201; responding to and following up with, 192; surveying, 191

Policies: human resources, understanding, 145

Political balance: developing, 106–8

Political climate: understanding, 113

Politics: organizational, new positions and, 234; playing politics the right way, 114–15

Population health management, 30

Porath, C., 242

Positive attitude: projecting, 32

Positive perception(s): constant and diverse feedback and, 18–19; earning, 21; effective communication and, 19–20; fostering, 16–20; modeling desired behavior and, 2; respect and, 17–18

Positive relationships: building, healthcare leadership and, 5

Positive tone: setting, 98–99

Power: being mindful of, 245; perks and imbalance of, 12

Praise: liberal use of, 33

Prejudice, 264

Preparation: effective verbal communication and, 169

Presentations: persuasive, 169

Presidential campaigns: racial and gender equality and, 259

Principles of Scientific Management, The (Taylor), 317, 318

Procedural justice methods: physician relationships and, 194

Professional advancement: workforce interactions and, 92

Professional code of ethics: adhering to, 63

Professional development plans: feedback and, 18

Professional image, 25–41; building, 28–29, 38–40; defining, 27; displaying appropriate demeanor, 31–33; dual impact of personal characteristics and group affiliations and, 34; enhancing, protocol for, *29;* "executive presence" and, 25; feedback about, 38; importance of, 26; maintaining professional style, 29–31; positive, characteristics contributing to, 27, *28;* professional reputation, personal and organizational results, and, *46;* professional reputation *versus,* 43, 45; self-reflection and, 38, 39–40; social media and, 37; strength of character and, 33–37

Professional life: personal life kept separate from, 244–45

Professional network: building, 107

Professional reputation, 43–56; building inside the organization, 51; building outside the organization, 50–51; communication and, 54; crafting your marketing

Professional reputation (*continued*)
strategy for, 49–51; developing,
45–47; earning, 43, 44; enhancing, protocol for, *47*; ethics and,
63; evolution of, 48; fragility of,
52; grounding in honesty and
integrity, 53, 55; implementing
and updating, 51–52; nurturing,
52–53; professional image, personal and organizational results,
and, *46*; professional image *versus*, 43, 45; relationship between
professional image and, *46*; self-
reflection and, 54; transparency
and, 54, 55; understanding your
current reputation, 47
Professional style. *See also* Professional
image: maintaining, 29–31
Progressive discipline: ethical human
resources decisions and, 148;
respect for employee and, 150
Promises: commitment and, 35; delivering on, 230
Promotion process: potential for
good fit and evaluative phase of,
234
Protocol(s): for appropriate office
etiquette, *243*; for candidates,
214; for candidate selection, *208*;
for developing a staff focus, *92*;
for effective board relations, *129*;
for effective office politics, *111*;
for effective use of technology in
communication, *173*; for effective
written communication, *170*; for
enhancing emotional intelligence,
74; for enhancing gender diversity, *266*; for enhancing professional image, *29*; for enhancing
professional reputation, *47*; for
enhancing racial, ethnic, and
cultural diversity, *263*; for ethical leadership, *61*; for executive
behavior, *17*, 17–20; for human
resources management, *144*; for
managing perception, *14*, 14–16;
for managing a multigenerational

workforce, *281*; for physician
business partnerships, *193*; for
physician customer service, *188*;
rich and deep meaning of word
itself, xxi; for success in new position, *226*; for verbal communication, *166*
Public advocacy: Affordable Care Act
and, 50–51
Punctuality: new role and, 227

Quality metrics: as public information,
126
Quality of care: governing board and,
127–28
Questions: active listening and, 304,
304; interview, being prepared
for, 216

Race: census data on, 258; compensa-
tion and, 260
Race relations: organizational, ACHE
survey results, 261, *261*
Racial discrimination, 260
Racial diversity: enhancing, 262–66,
263
Racial equality: 2008 presidential cam-
paign and, 259
*Racial/Ethnic Comparison of Career
Attainment in Healthcare Manage-
ment, A,* 259
Racial tensions: open dialogue and,
263–64
Raskin, R., 300
Reality: perception *versus*, 4–5
"Reality and rhetoric" gap: understand-
ing and reducing, 22
Recession of 2007–2009: executive
compensation issue and, 11
Recruitment: competitive compensa-
tion and, 151; honoring confiden-
tiality and, 210–11; poor, costly
hiring mistakes and, 205; vast
implications tied to, 217
Reductions in workforce, 143
Reference checking: confidentiality
and, 211

Reflection, 304; self-awareness and, 299; taking time for, 296
Regulations: human resources, knowing, 144–46, 156
Regulatory compliance: organizational code of ethics and, 62
Reimbursement: ethical human resources decisions and, 146
Relationship building, leadership success and, 80–81
Relationship equity: positive, 31–32
Release-of-liability form: termination and, 150
Reputation. See Professional reputation
Resignations, 154
Respect, 37; building relationships based on, 115; courtesy and, 32; demonstrating, guidelines for, 149–51; demonstrating at all times, 17–18; diversity and, 262; gender diversity and, 266; for governing board members, 137; inclusiveness and, 262; multigenerational workforce and, 276–78, 286; new role and, 235; office etiquette and, 246; for physicians, 189–90, 197; time constraints, professional sociability, and, 248
Retained search arrangement: executive search firms and, 211
Retention, 143, 154
Retirement: baby boomers and glide path to, 283
Retreats, 296
Reynolds, Britt T., 53–55
Risk: physician relationships and, 194
Roberto, M. A., 106
Roberts, L. M., 34
Romantic relationships, 268
Rotary Club, 50
Rounding: interpersonal connections and, 76
Rude behavior, 31, 242
Rules of engagement: setting up, 115–16
Rumors, 243

Salaries: operating expenses and, 142; pay equity issues and, 268; understanding nuances of, 151–52
Schermerhorn, J. R., 64
Schwarzkopf, Norman: on leadership, 36
Scientific management: evolution of, 318–20
Scientific management theory (Taylor), 318
Scope of responsibility: jealousy and, 109
Screening: of board members, 130
Securities and Exchange Commission (SEC): executive compensation and, 11
Selection. See Candidate selection
Selection assessment model, 212, 213
Selection practices: poor, costly hiring mistakes and, 205
Self-awareness, 10; avoiding managerial derailment and, 233; career derailments and lack of, 16; challenges in, 300–302; components of, 296–99, 297; concerted focus on, 304; critical role of, in leaders' growth and development, 295; definition of, 300; emotional intelligence and, 73, 74, 293; enhancing, methods for, 302–6; feedback and, 18–19; framing in objective descriptors, 297, 298; improving, 75–76; inappropriate office behavior and lack of, 243; increased level of, performance, and, 7; inverse relationship between derailment and, 309–10, 310; leadership success and, 295; learning from weaknesses, 299–300; low feeding even lower, 301; seeing yourself as others do, 301–2; strategic view of, 302–3; success and, 295, 296; tips for, 294–95, 311
Self-concept, 297
Self-esteem, 297
Selfishness: unethical behavior and, 63

Verbal communication (*continued*)
practice dialogue, not monologue
in, 166–67; preparation and, 169;
protocol for, *166*
Vietnam War, 279
Visibility: maintaining, 22; new role
and, 227
Vision statement: diversity included
in, 263
Voicemails: *New York Times* test and,
175

Wal-Mart: executive compensation at,
11
Wan, K. E., 307
Watkins, Michael C., 223
Watsabaugh, D., 307
Weaknesses: learning from, 299–300
Weight maintenance: professional
image and, 31
Wellness: promoting, 30–31
Whitehead, J., 298
Win–win, learning art of, 117
Women: baby boomer, large initial
influx into workforce, *281*; in
healthcare leadership, 259–60; pay
equity issues and, 268; presiden-
tial candidates, 259; work and

family commitments and, 268–69;
work–life balance and, 260
Work and family commitments: supporting balance between, 268–69
Work ethic: of baby boomers, 279,
281, 282–83; of generation X,
279–80, *281,* 284–85; of millennials, 280, *281,* 285; of silent
generation, 279, *281*; strong,
demonstrating, 32
Workforce management: operating
expenses and, 142
Workforce quality: competitive advantage through, 156
Work–life balance: gender and, 260;
generation X and, 283–84
World War II, 279, 282
Written communication: advantages
and risks with, 169; clear, personal
style in, 171–72; effective, 169–72;
handwritten notes, 172; mental
checklist for, 170–71; protocol for,
170; selectivity in, 170; timing of,
171

YouTube, 177

Zenger, J., 298

About the Authors

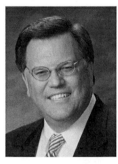

Carson F. Dye, FACHE, president and CEO of Exceptional Leadership, LLC, is a seasoned leadership consultant with more than 40 years of leadership and management experience. Over the past 20 years, he has conducted hundreds of leadership searches for healthcare organizations, helping to fill CEO, COO, CFO, and physician executive roles in health systems, academic medical centers, universities, and free-standing hospitals.

Dye has provided clients with extensive counsel in succession and transition planning, executive leadership assessment, CEO evaluation, coaching, and retreat facilitation. He is certified to use the Hogan Leadership Assessment tests for evaluation, coaching, and leadership development. He also has extensive experience working with physician leaders and has helped organizations establish physician leadership development programs.

Dye has served as an executive search consultant and partner with Witt/Kieffer, TMP Worldwide, and LAI/Lamalie Associates. Earlier, he was partner and director of Findley Davies's healthcare consulting division in Toledo, Ohio. Dye has had 20 years of experience in healthcare administration, serving in executive-level positions at St. Vincent Mercy Medical Center in Toledo; the Ohio State University Medical Center in Columbus; and Children's

Hospital Medical Center and Clermont Mercy Hospital, both in Cincinnati.

Dye has been a regular faculty member for the American College of Healthcare Executives (ACHE) since 1987 and has presented workshops for about 40 state and local hospital associations. He also teaches in the ACHE Board of Governors Examination prep course. In addition, Dye is a faculty member of the Governance Institute and currently holds a faculty appointment at the University of Alabama-Birmingham in its executive master's program. Dye has written nine previous books, all with Health Administration Press, including two James A. Hamilton Book of the Year winners, *Developing Physician Leaders for Successful Clinical Integration* (2013) and *Leadership in Healthcare: Values at the Top* (2000). His other titles include *Exceptional Leadership: 16 Critical Competencies for Healthcare Executives*, second edition (2015); *Leadership in Healthcare: Essential Values and Skills*, second edition (2010); *Winning the Talent War* (2002); and *Protocols for Healthcare Executive Behavior* (1993). The Dye–Garman Leadership Competency Model, from *Exceptional Leadership*, has been used by many healthcare organizations as a competency model for assessment, executive selection, development, and succession planning.

Dye earned his bachelor's degree from Marietta College and his master of business administration degree from Xavier University.

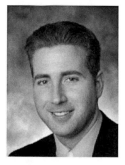 **Brett D. Lee, PhD, FACHE,** currently serves as a market chief executive officer for Tenet Healthcare. In this role, he oversees the operations and strategic planning for several acute care hospitals, an expansive ambulatory enterprise, and an employed multispecialty physician group providing care to communities in northern and eastern Texas.

Lee has spent 15 years in healthcare as a clinician, a clinical leader, and an executive. He has spent the majority of his career in pediatric healthcare, serving in executive roles at four of the nation's ten largest children's hospitals. Lee is the lead author of the best-selling book *Growing Leaders in Healthcare: Lessons from the Corporate World* (Health Administration Press, 2009) and the subsequent American College of Healthcare Executives self-study course *Creating a Leadership Development Program in Your Healthcare Organization.* He also wrote a second book, *Managing Clinically: What Can Medicine Teach Us About Leadership?* (America Star Books, 2011).

Lee holds a bachelor of science degree in physical therapy from the University of Oklahoma, a master of health science degree in health finance and management from the Johns Hopkins School of Public Health, a master of science in leadership development degree from the University of Pennsylvania Wharton School of Business, a doctorate in allied health from the Massachusetts General Hospital Institute of Health Professions, and a doctor of philosophy degree in executive leadership from Louisiana Baptist University.

In 2011, Lee received the Robert S. Hudgens Memorial Award for Young Healthcare Executive of the Year from the American College of Healthcare Executives. He also was recognized as a "Rising Star" of the healthcare industry by *Becker's Hospital Review* in 2012, 2013, and 2014 and as an "Up and Comer" by *Modern Healthcare* in 2013. In 2014, the *Dallas Business Journal* included Lee in its "Who's Who in Healthcare."